INTERVENTIONAL CARDIOLOGY CLINICS

www.interventional.theclinics.com

Editor-in-Chief

MARVIN H. ENG

Mechanical Circulatory Support

April 2021 • Volume 10 • Number 2

Editor

BRIAN O'NEILL

ELSEVIER

1600 John F. Kennedy Boulevard • Suite 1800 • Philadelphia, Pennsylvania, 19103-2899

http://www.theclinics.com

INTERVENTIONAL CARDIOLOGY CLINICS Volume 10, Number 2
April 2021 ISSN 2211-7458, ISBN-13: 978-0-323-81323-5

Editor: Joanna Collett
Developmental Editor: Donald Mumford

Interventional Cardiology Clinics (ISSN 2211-7458) is published quarterly by Elsevier Inc., 360 Park Avenue South, New York, NY 10010-1710. Months of issue are January, April, July, and October. Subscription prices are USD 209 per year for US individuals, USD 622 for US institutions, USD 100 per year for US students, USD 209 per year for Canadian individuals, USD 638 for Canadian institutions, USD 100 per year for Canadian students, USD 296 per year for international individuals, USD 638 for international institutions, and USD 150 per year for international students. To receive student/resident rate, orders must be accompanied by name of affiliated institution, date of term, and the *signature* of program/residency coordinator on institution letterhead. Orders will be billed at individual rate until proof of status is received. Foreign air speed delivery is included in all *Clinics* subscription prices. All prices are subject to change without notice. **POSTMASTER:** Send address changes to *Interventional Cardiology Clinics*, Elsevier Health Sciences Division, Subscription Customer Service, 3251 Riverport Lane, Maryland Heights, MO 63043. **Customer Service: Telephone: 1-800-654-2452** (U.S. and Canada); **1-314-447-8871** (outside U.S. and Canada). **Fax: 1-314-447-8029. E-mail: journalscustomerservice-usa@elsevier.com (for print support); journalsonlinesupport-usa@elsevier.com (for online support).**

Reprints. For copies of 100 or more of articles in this publication, please contact the Commercial Reprints Department, Elsevier Inc., 360 Park Avenue South, New York, NY 10010-1710. Tel.: 212-633-3874; Fax: 212-633-3820; E-mail: reprints@elsevier.com.

CONTRIBUTORS

CONSULTING EDITOR

MARVIN H. ENG, MD
Director of Research for the Center of
Structural Heart Disease, Structural Heart
Disease Fellowship Director, Henry Ford
Hospital, Department of Structural Heart
Disease, Division of Cardiology, Henry Ford
Health System, Detroit, Michigan, USA

EDITOR

BRIAN O'NEILL, MD, FACC
Center for Structural Heart Disease, Henry
Ford Hospital, Department of Structural Heart
Disease, Division of Cardiology, Henry Ford
Health System, Detroit, Michigan, USA

AUTHORS

VIKAS AGGARWAL, MD, MPH
Assistant Professor of Clinical Medicine,
Division of Cardiology, Department of Internal
Medicine, University of Michigan Medical
School, Ann Arbor, Michigan, USA

AKBARSHAKH AKHMEROV, MD
Post-doctoral Research Fellow, Department of
Cardiac Surgery, Smidt Heart Institute,
Cedars-Sinai Medical Center, Los Angeles,
California, USA

KHALDOON ALASWAD, MD
Director of Cardiac Catheterization
Laboratories, Interventional Cardiology, Henry
Ford Hospital, Detroit, Michigan, USA

SONALI ARORA, MD
Institute of Heart and Lung Transplant, Krishna
Institute of Medical Sciences Hospitals,
Secunderabad, Telangana, India

AURAS R. ATREYA, MD
Interventional Cardiology, AIG Institute of
Cardiac Sciences and Research, Hyderabad,
Telangana, India

MIR B. BASIR, DO, FACC, FSCAI
Henry Ford Health Care System, Director,
STEMI, Director, Acute Mechanical Circulatory
Support, Interventional Cardiology, Senior

Staff, Henry Ford Hospital, Detroit, Michigan,
USA

EDO Y. BIRATI, MD
Assistant Professor, Division of Cardiovascular
Medicine, University of Pennsylvania,
Philadelphia, Pennsylvania, USA; Division of
Cardiovascular Medicine, Poriya Medical
Center, Israel; Perelman Center for Advanced
Medicine, Philadelphia, Pennsylvania, USA

YEVGENIY BRAILOVSKY, DO, MSc
Assistant Professor, Division of Cardiology,
Department of Medicine, Sidney Kimmel
School of Medicine, Thomas Jefferson
University, Philadelphia, Pennsylvania, USA

AMY E. CHENEY, MD
Acting Clinical Instructor, Department of
Internal Medicine, Division of Cardiology,
University of Washington Medical Center,
Seattle, Washington, USA

MOHAMMED FERRAS DABBAGH, MD
Fellow in Cardiovascular Medicine, Division of
Cardiology, Henry Ford Hospital, Detroit,
Michigan, USA

MARVIN H. ENG, MD
Director of Research for the Center of
Structural Heart Disease, Structural Heart

Disease Fellowship Director, Henry Ford Hospital, Department of Structural Heart Disease, Division of Cardiology, Henry Ford Health System, Detroit, Michigan, USA

TIBERIO FRISOLI, MD
Department of Structural Heart Disease, Division of Cardiology, Henry Ford Health System, Detroit, Michigan, USA

TYLER M. GUNN, MD
Division of Cardiothoracic Surgery, University of Kentucky, Lexington, Kentucky, USA

JOHN C. GURLEY, MD
Division of Cardiovascular Medicine, University of Kentucky, Gill Heart and Vascular Institute, Lexington, Kentucky, USA

AMIR KAKI, MD
Division of Interventional Cardiology, Department of Medicine, Ascension St John Hospital, Detroit, Michigan, USA

SURESH KESHAVAMURTHY, MD, FACS, FRCS
Division of Cardiothoracic Surgery, University of Kentucky, Lexington, Kentucky, USA

KATHERINE J. KUNKEL, MD, MSEd
Fellow in Complex, High-Risk and Indicated Coronary Interventions and Advanced Hemodynamic Care (CHIP), Interventional Cardiology, Henry Ford Hospital, Detroit, Michigan, USA

VLADIMIR LAKHTER, DO
Division of Cardiovascular Diseases, Department of Medicine, Temple University Hospital, Lewis Katz School of Medicine, Philadelphia, Pennsylvania, USA

JAMES LEE, MD
Department of Structural Heart Disease, Division of Cardiology, Henry Ford Health System, Detroit, Michigan, USA

ALEJANDRO LEMOR, MD, MSc
Department of Structural Heart Disease, Division of Cardiology, Henry Ford Health System, Detroit, Michigan, USA

RAJASEKHAR S.R. MALYALA, MD
Division of Cardiothoracic Surgery, University of Kentucky, Lexington, Kentucky, USA

JAMES M. McCABE, MD
Associate Professor, Section Chief Interventional Cardiology, Department of Internal Medicine, Division of Cardiology, University of Washington Medical Center, Seattle, Washington, USA

STEPHEN McHUGH, MD
Department of Medicine, Temple University Hospital, Lewis Katz School of Medicine, Philadelphia, Pennsylvania, USA

SURAJ MISHRA, MD
Department of Medicine, Temple University Hospital, Lewis Katz School of Medicine, Philadelphia, Pennsylvania, USA

PAUL NONA, MD
Department of Structural Heart Disease, Division of Cardiology, Henry Ford Health System, Detroit, Michigan, USA

ALI NOORY, MD
Department of Medicine, Temple University Hospital, Lewis Katz School of Medicine, Philadelphia, Pennsylvania, USA

BRIAN O'NEILL, MD, FACC
Center for Structural Heart Disease, Henry Ford Hospital, Department of Structural Heart Disease, Division of Cardiology, Henry Ford Health System, Detroit, Michigan, USA

WILLIAM W. O'NEILL, MD
Department of Structural Heart Disease, Division of Cardiology, Henry Ford Health System, Detroit, Michigan, USA

ESTEFANIA OLIVEROS, MD, MSc
Assistant Professor, Division of Cardiology, Department of Medicine, Temple University Hospital, Lewis Katz School of Medicine, Philadelphia, Pennsylvania, USA

MOHAMMED QINTAR, MD, MSc
Department of Structural Heart Disease, Division of Cardiology, Henry Ford Health System, Detroit, Michigan, USA

DANNY RAMZY, MD, PhD
Director of Robotic Cardiac Surgery, Director of Lung Transplantation, Interim Director of MCS, Department of Cardiac Surgery, Smidt Heart Institute, Cedars-Sinai Medical Center, Los Angeles, California, USA

SUPRIYA SHORE, MD, MSCS
Clinical Lecturer, Department of Internal
Medicine, Division of Cardiovascular Disease,
University of Michigan, Ann Arbor, Michigan,
USA

HEMINDERMEET SINGH, MD
Division of Cardiology, Department of
Medicine, Mercy-Health St Vincent Medical
Center, Toledo, Ohio, USA

SUMIT SOHAL, MD
Division of Cardiovascular Diseases,
Department of Medicine, RWJ Barnabas
Heath Newark Beth Israel Medical Center,
Newark, New Jersey, USA

RAJIV TAYAL, MD, MPH, FACC, FSCAI
Division of Cardiovascular Diseases,
Department of Medicine, RWJ Barnabas
Heath Newark Beth Israel Medical Center,
Newark, New Jersey, USA

CATHERINE VANCHIERE, MD
Department of Medicine, Temple University
Hospital, Lewis Katz School of Medicine,
Philadelphia, Pennsylvania, USA

PEDRO VILLABLANCA, MD, MSc
Department of Structural Heart Disease,
Division of Cardiology, Henry Ford Health
System, Detroit, Michigan, USA

DEE DEE WANG, MD
Department of Structural Heart Disease,
Division of Cardiology, Henry Ford Health
System, Detroit, Michigan, USA

LINA YA'QOUB, MD
Louisiana State University, One University
Place, Shreveport, Louisiana, USA

MOHAMMAD ZAIDAN, MD
Interventional Cardiology, Henry Ford
Hospital, Detroit, Michigan, USA

CONTENTS

Overview of Options for Mechanical Circulatory Support   **147**
Estefania Oliveros, Yevgeniy Brailovsky, and Vikas Aggarwal

> Mechanical circulatory support is used widely in acute setting of myocardial infarction, myocarditis, and cardiogenic shock as well as in chronic scenarios with advanced end-stage heart failure. Different algorithmic approaches can help the clinician decide the type of support required in a high morbidity and mortality setting. It is paramount to emphasize the need for a multidisciplinary approach to make steadfast decisions in the acute settings of cardiogenic shock.

Vascular Access for Large Bore Access   **157**
Stephen McHugh, Ali Noory, Suraj Mishra, Catherine Vanchiere, and Vladimir Lakhter

> Recent advances in the field of interventional cardiology have allowed for more complex procedures to be performed percutaneously. Ability to obtain safe large bore vascular access is frequently the key factor to procedural success. Meticulous technique for successful vascular access incorporates the understanding of anatomic landmarks, ultrasound, fluoroscopy, and micropuncture. Adequate hemostasis at the end of the case can be achieved through careful use of commercially available vascular closure devices. Although access-related vascular complications are uncommon, early recognition is key to successful management. Arterial tortuosity and calcification can present a significant challenge to successful common femoral artery access.

Mechanical Circulatory Support in Acute Myocardial Infarction and Cardiogenic Shock   **169**
Alejandro Lemor, Lina Ya'qoub, and Mir B. Basir

> Mechanical circulatory support devices are increasingly used for the treatment of acute myocardial infarction complicated by cardiogenic shock. These devices provide different levels of univentricular and biventricular support, have different mechanisms of actions, and provide different physiologic effects. Institutions require expert teams to safely implant and manage these devices. This article reviews the mechanism of action, physiologic effects, and data as they relate to the utilization of these devices.

Mechanical Circulatory Support in Right Ventricular Failure   **185**
Akbarshakh Akhmerov and Danny Ramzy

> Right ventricular dysfunction presents unique challenges in patients with cardiopulmonary disease. When optimal medical therapy fails, mechanical circulatory support is considered. Devices can by classified according to whether they are deployed percutaneously or surgically, whether the pump is axial or centrifugal, whether the right ventricle is bypassed directly or indirectly, and whether the support is short term or long term. Each device has advantages and disadvantages. Acute mechanical circulatory support is a suitable temporizing strategy in advanced heart failure. Future research in right ventricular mechanical circulatory support will optimize device management, refine patient selection, and ultimately improve clinical outcomes.

The prevalence of extracorporeal cardiopulmonary resuscitation is increasing worldwide as more health care centers develop the necessary infrastructure, protocols, and technical expertise required to provide mobile extracorporeal life support with short notice. Strict adherence to patient selection guidelines in the setting of out-of-hospital cardiac arrest, as well as in-hospital cardiac arrest, allows for improved survival with neurologically favorable outcomes in a larger patient population. This review discusses the preferred approaches, cannulation techniques, and available support devices ideal for the various clinical situations encountered during the treatment of cardiac arrest and refractory cardiogenic shock.

The use of mechanical circulatory devices to support high-risk elective percutaneous coronary intervention (PCI) has become more common as the group of patients considered inoperable or high risk for surgical revascularization has grown. Most of the data examining outcomes in high-risk PCI are observational and retrospective. Limited prospective randomized studies have been unable to show improved clinical outcomes with routine mechanical circulatory support (MCS) in patients with a high burden of coronary artery disease and reduced ejection fraction. The role for MCS in high-risk PCI continues to evolve as understanding of the appropriate groups for this therapy evolves.

Despite advances in cardiovascular care, managing cardiogenic shock caused by structural heart disease is challenging. Patients with cardiogenic shock are critically ill upon presentation and require early disease recognition and rapid escalation of care. Temporary mechanical circulatory support provides a higher level of care than current medical therapies such as vasopressors and inotropes. This review article focuses on the role of hemodynamic monitoring, mechanical circulatory support, and device selection in patients who present with cardiogenic shock due to structural heart disease. Early initiation of appropriate mechanical circulatory support may reduce morbidity and mortality.

Advanced heart failure refractory to medical therapy can result in patients presenting with progressively worsening hypoperfusion and cardiogenic shock. Temporary mechanical circulatory support is often necessary as a bridge to heart transplant or durable ventricular assist devices. These devices increase cardiac output. Several options are available for left ventricular support. With the exception of venoarterial extracorporeal membrane oxygenation, all other devices decrease left ventricular end-diastolic pressure. The choice of device should be driven by patient needs and the treating teams comfort. Timely identification of cardiogenic shock and use of shock teams are potential strategies that can help improve survival.

Large Sheath Management in Patients with Poor Peripheral Access   251
Amir Kaki and Hemindermeet Singh

Despite the evolution of device technology and increasing operator experience, vascular and bleeding complications remain a major source of perioperative morbidity and mortality, particularly in patients with peripheral arterial disease. These complications may be compounded with the use of large bore access sheaths for mechanical support, which may be required to be left in the vessels for a prolonged period of time. Through this article, the authors demonstrate the importance of assessment for peripheral arterial disease before insertion of large bore sheaths. They also describe various strategies to manage occlusive sheaths for distal reperfusion and percutaneous axillary artery access as an alternate option.

Alternative Access for Mechanical Circulatory Support   257
Amy E. Cheney and James M. McCabe

Femoral arterial access is the default strategy for large-bore interventional procedures, including temporary mechanical circulatory support implantation and structural heart therapies, based on superior outcomes and operator ease. In addition to patient size and comorbidities, vessel tortuosity, significant calcification, and diminutive vessel caliber all may make iliofemoral access prohibitively high risk or impossible. Given the increase of large-bore transcatheter procedures, bleeding avoidance strategies are essential and thus novel mechanisms for large-bore access have evolved. This article highlights the advantages, limitations, and practical approaches to the 2 most common percutaneous large-bore alternative access strategies: transaxillary and transcaval access.

Mechanical Circulatory Support Devices: Management and Prevention of   269
Vascular Complications
Sumit Sohal and Rajiv Tayal

The use of mechanical circulatory support devices has seen a dramatic rise over the last few years owing to their increased use not only in acute circulatory collapse but also their prophylactic use in high-risk procedures. These devices continue to have their overall benefits marginalized due to the relatively high rates of complications. Vascular complications are the most common and are associated with increased risk of mortality in these patients. Preventive measures at each stage of procedure, frequent monitoring and assessment to recognize early signs of deterioration are the best ways to mitigate the effects of vascular complications.

MECHANICAL CIRCULATORY SUPPORT

RELATED SERIES

Cardiology Clinics
https://www.cardiology.theclinics.com/
Cardiac Electrophysiology Clinics
https://www.cardiacep.theclinics.com/
Heart Failure Clinics
https://www.heartfailure.theclinics.com/

THE CLINICS ARE NOW AVAILABLE ONLINE!

Access your subscription at:
www.theclinics.com

FOREWORD

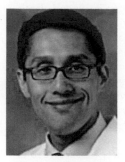

Marvin H. Eng, MD
Consulting Editor

We are pleased to introduce this issue of *Interventional Cardiology Clinics* detailing the use of mechanical circulatory support (MCS) for cardiogenic shock. In pace with much of interventional cardiology, management of cardiogenic shock has been a key area of growth in the past decade. Leaps in MCS devices and large-bore access management have rapidly advanced the field of cardiogenic shock.

Recent years have seen the rising utilization of a variety of MCS devices in the cardiac catheterization laboratory. For a generation, intra-aortic balloon pumps were the chief tools of circulatory support available for cardiologists, and for decades, the mortality rate in cardiogenic shock was on a plateaued trajectory. With the advent of a percutaneous axial flow pump, the Impella (Abiomed, Danvers, MA, USA), and improving familiarity with managing large-bore access, clinicians have been increasingly aggressive with treating cardiogenic shock. As the limits of initial versions of the Impella were tested, clinicians found the need to escalate the level of MCS provided. Devices such as the extracorporeal membrane oxygenation and the Tandem Heart (LivaNova PLC, London, UK) entered the repertoire of interventional cardiologists, and a more diverse set of tools for treating both left and right ventricular failure are now being used. Fueled by the improvements in MCS and vascular access, the needle in cardiogenic shock mortality has finally moved in a positive direction.

This issue of *Interventional Cardiology Clinics* has been edited by Dr Brian P. O'Neill, a fierce advocate and leader in improving cardiogenic shock outcomes. We congratulate him on assembling the latest in MCS and vascular access management strategies. Expect to find the issue comprehensive and enlightening.

Marvin H. Eng, MD
Center of Structural Heart Disease
Henry Ford Hospital
Clara Ford Pavilion RM 434
2799 West Grand Boulevard
Detroit, MI 48202, USA

E-mail address:
meng1@hfhs.org

Intervent Cardiol Clin 10 (2021) xi
https://doi.org/10.1016/j.iccl.2021.02.002
2211-7458/21/© 2021 Published by Elsevier Inc.

PREFACE

Mechanical Circulatory Support

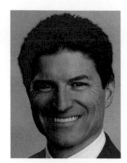

Brian O'Neill, MD, FACC
Editor

The utilization of mechanical circulatory support (MCS) has increased in the United States over the past 10 years. MCS initially primarily consisted of the intra-aortic balloon pump and surgical implantation of extracorporeal membrane oxygenation, but there are now an ever-increasing number of devices with unique characteristics in terms of the amount of hemodynamic support provided, as well as the option for isolated right- and left-sided support. Moving forward from the need for surgical cutdowns for the implantation of these large-bore devices, the routine use of ultrasound-guided access with small-gauge micropuncture needles has facilitated the transformation of these procedures to a totally percutaneous one. The field of structural heart disease has helped to usher in this era with the need for reliable access and closure of large-bore access to allow delivery of transcatheter aortic valve replacement therapy.

As many patients have peripheral arterial disease, we continue to seek out new techniques to allow perfusion to the leg during hemodynamic support, and to be able to better manage vascular complications when they may occur. In those patients who are eligible, the use of vascular closure devices has allowed for the safe explant during the same setting or on a different day when the device is no longer required.

We have come to realize the importance of MCS outside of those patients solely with cardiogenic shock. The fields of high-risk percutaneous coronary intervention and structural heart disease have benefited from the advances in MCS to allow us to treat these higher-risk patients who may not have been candidates for anything before. We have also now gained more experience in intermediate-term MCS for those patients who may require a long-term durable ventricular assist device or heart transplant. In this issue of *Interventional Cardiology Clinics*, we hope to touch on each of these issues and offer a single source of information for those who have an interest in MCS. On behalf of my coauthors, we hope you enjoy the issue.

Brian O'Neill, MD, FACC
Center of Structural Heart Disease
Henry Ford Hospital
Clara Ford Pavillion Room 440
Detroit, MI 48202, USA

E-mail address:
bpoatumich@yahoo.com

Intervent Cardiol Clin 10 (2021) xiii
https://doi.org/10.1016/j.iccl.2021.02.001

PREFACE

Mechanical Circulatory Support

Brian O'Neill, MD, FACC
Editor

The utilization of mechanical circulatory support (MCS) has increased in the United States over the past 10 years. MCS initially primarily consisted of the intra-aortic balloon pump and surgical implantation of extracorporeal membrane oxygenation, but there are now an ever-increasing number of devices with unique characteristics in terms of the amount of hemodynamic support provided, as well as the option for isolated right and left-sided support. Moving forward from the need for surgical cutdowns for the implantation of these large-bore devices, the routine use of ultrasound-guided access with small-gauge micro-puncture needles has facilitated the transformation of these procedures to a totally percutaneous one. The field of structural heart disease has helped to usher in the era with the need for reliable access and closure of large-bore access to allow delivery of transcatheter aortic valve replacement therapy.

As many patients have peripheral arterial disease, we continue to seek out new techniques to allow perfusion to the leg during hemodynamic support, and to be able to better manage vascular complications when they may occur. In those patients who are eligible, the use of vascular closure devices has allowed for the safe explant during the same setting or on a different day when the device is no longer required.

We have come to realize the importance of MCS outside of those patients solely with cardiogenic shock. The fields of high-risk percutaneous coronary intervention and structural heart disease have benefited from the advances in MCS to allow us to treat these higher-risk patients who may not have been candidates for anything before. We have also now gained more experience in intermediate-term MCS for those patients who may require a long-term durable ventricular assist device or heart transplant. In this issue of Interventional Cardiology Clinics, we hope to touch on each of these issues and offer a single source of information for those who have an interest in MCS. On behalf of my coauthors, we hope you enjoy the issue.

Brian O'Neill, MD, FACC
Center of Structural Heart Disease
Henry Ford Hospital
Clara Ford Pavilion Room 440
Detroit, MI 48202, USA

E-mail address:
boneill2@hfhs.org

Intervent Cardiol Clin 10 (2021) xiii
https://doi.org/10.1016/j.iccl.2021.02.001
2211-7458/21/© 2021 Published by Elsevier Inc.

Overview of Options for Mechanical Circulatory Support

Estefania Oliveros, MD, MSc[a],
Yevgeniy Brailovsky, DO, MSc[b],
Vikas Aggarwal, MD, MPH[c],*

KEYWORDS

• Mechanical circulatory support • Heart failure • Cardiogenic shock

KEY POINTS

- Mechanical circulatory support is used widely in acute setting of myocardial infarction, myocarditis, and cardiogenic shock as well as in chronic scenarios with advanced end-stage heart failure.
- Different algorithmic approaches can help the clinician decide the type of support required in a high morbidity and mortality setting.
- It is paramount to emphasize the need for a multidisciplinary approach to make steadfast decisions in the acute settings of cardiogenic shock.

INTRODUCTION

According to the American Heart Association, approximately 6.1 million people have heart failure (HF) in the United States. Of those individuals, 10% have advanced end-stage HF.[1] Unfortunately, projections suggest that the prevalence of HF will increase by 46% from 2012 to 2030, resulting in more than 8 million people greater than or equal to18 years of age with HF.[2]

The term, *advanced HF*, signifies individuals with circulatory insufficiency leading to HF symptoms with minimal exertion or at rest, recurrent decompensation, and severe cardiac dysfunction.[3] The term, advanced HF, includes acute cardiogenic shock and refractory stage D HF patients. Cardiogenic shock occurs in more than 8% of myocardial infarctions and is associated with a mortality of approximately 50%,[4,5] whereas refractory stage D HF has up to 80% 5-year

mortality rate.[6] For stage D patients or advanced end-stage HF patients, who are appropriate candidates, heart transplantation remains the treatment of choice and offers the best quality of life and longest life. Moreover, heart transplantation has a 1-year survival of 87% and a 10-year survival of 50%.[7] There is a substantial shortage of organs, however, and only approximately 3552 heart transplants were performed in 2019 nationwide.[8] Therefore, in the context of a prevalent and increasing HF population and a shortage of heart donors, mechanical circulatory support (MCS) has emerged as a way to prolong survival and improve the quality of life in this very sick cohort by restoring organ hypoperfusion.[9] This article discusses MCS, including its history and indications, and describes the different devices available for it. An algorithmic approach to selecting adequate therapies in different complex cardiovascular scenarios also is provided.

[a] Division of Cardiology, Department of Medicine, Lewis Katz School of Medicine, Temple University Hospital, 3401 North Broad Street, Philadelphia, PA 19140, USA; [b] Division of Cardiology, Department of Medicine, Sidney Kimmel School of Medicine, Thomas Jefferson University, 833 Chestnut Street, Suite 640, Philadelphia, PA 19107, USA; [c] Division of Cardiology, Department of Internal Medicine, University of Michigan Medical School, 1500 East Medical Center Drive, SPC 5869, Ann Arbor, MI 48109, USA
* Corresponding author.
E-mail address: aggarwav@med.umich.edu

Intervent Cardiol Clin 10 (2021) 147–156
https://doi.org/10.1016/j.iccl.2020.12.009
2211-7458/21/© 2021 Elsevier Inc. All rights reserved.

HISTORY OF MECHANICAL CIRCULATORY SUPPORT

The development of cardiopulmonary bypass and open heart surgery brought interest in MCS. On May 6, 1953, Dr John H Gibbon, Jr, completed the first successful procedure with the heart-lung machine, which consisted of an atrial septal defect closure.[10] It was a proof of concept. Simultaneously, Dr Michael E. DeBakey developed the first blood pump as a medical student, then continued to work in this field, and in 1963 became the first to use a ventricular assist device (VAD).[11] DeBakey used a gas-energized double-lumen silastic tube reinforced with Dacron connected from the left atrium (LA) to the descending aorta. These advances led to the first successful left VAD (LVAD) as a bridge to recovery (BTR) in 1966.[12] Subsequently, the National Heart, Lung, and Blood Institute; industry; biomedical engineers; cardiologists; and cardiothoracic surgeons collaborated to develop LVADs and a total artificial heart. Finally, in 1982, Dr Barney Clark was the first patient to receive the Food and Drug Administration (FDA)-approved Jarvik-7 total artificial heart as a destination device.[13] In 1985, the first successful bridge to transplant (BTT) took place.[14] A year later, the FDA approved the total artificial heart and other LVADs as BTTs. Across the United States, many surgeons did not have access to newer implantable devices. Therefore, short-term support devices were used in patients who could not be weaned off the heart-lung machine using centrifugal pumps.

The landmark Randomized Evaluation of Mechanical Assistance for the Treatment of Congestive Heart Failure (REMATCH) trial validated a 48% reduction in mortality among patients receiving a first-generation LVAD instead of optimal medical management.[15] Therefore, the FDA approved LVAD as destination therapy. Since then, there has been a steady evolution of MCS technology, from initial generations of pulsatile devices, to continuous flow devices,[16] to fully magnetically levitated continuous flow devices.[17,18] MCS use has become part of the management guidelines for advanced HF.

INDICATIONS FOR MECHANICAL CIRCULATORY SUPPORT

- Bridge to decision (BTD)/bridge to bridge (BTB): short-term MCS in cardiogenic shock cases until stabilization of end-organ perfusion or durable support options are considered. Contraindications for long-term MCS (eg, cerebral injury after resuscitation) are excluded. Additional therapeutic options, including long-term VAD therapy and heart transplant, can be considered.
- Bridge to candidacy (BTC): MCS (usually LVAD) improves end-organ function to make an ineligible patient eligible for heart transplantation.
- BTT: MCS (LVAD or biventricular VAD) keeps a patient who otherwise is at high risk of death alive until an organ donor becomes available.
- BTR: MCS (usually LVAD) keeps the patient alive until cardiac functioning recovers sufficiently to remove MCS.
- Destination therapy: long-term use of MCS as an alternative to transplantation in patients with advanced end-stage HF ineligible for transplantation or long-term waiting for heart transplantation

STRATIFICATION OF SEVERITY IN ADVANCED HEART FAILURE

There is no simple answer to the question of when MCS support is indicated. A risk-benefit assessment must be made. Therefore, patient-specific factors (age, body mass index anatomic features, prior sternotomies, comorbidities, and so forth), institutional experience, device availability, and acuity determine the support chosen. In general, the choice to use MCS support is based on the severity of HF. Hence, risk scores are valuable tools for grading the severity of disease, such as destination therapy[19] risk, and predicting RV failure.[20] These scores include HeartMate II,[21] the Seattle Heart Failure Model of survival,[22] Interagency Registry for Mechanically Assisted Circulatory Support (INTERMACS) classifications,[23] Society of Cardiovascular Angiography and Interventions (SCAI) classifications, Pulmonary Embolism Severity Index score,[24] Model for End-Stage Liver Disease score,[25] and Acute Physiology and Chronic Health Evaluation (APACHE) II.[26] None of these measures is used across all institutions.

INTERMACS profiles are used to stratify patients with HF in the New York Heart Association (NYHA) functional class III or class IV into 7 distinct profiles with increasing risks of mortality[27] (Table 1). Additional modifiers—such as arrhythmia, temporary circulatory support, and frequent flyer—are included in the initial design of the INTERMACS to characterize each group further. More recently, the expert consensus statement by SCAI presented a new integrative approach to further classifying patients with

Table 1
Interagency Registry for Mechanically Assisted Circulatory Support: profiles

Profiles	Description	Time Frame to Intervention
1	Critical cardiogenic shock	Within hours
2	Progressive decline on inotropic support	Within few days
3	Stable but inotrope dependent	Elective intervention over weeks to months
4	Resting symptoms home on oral therapy	Elective intervention over weeks to months
5	Exertion intolerant	Variable urgency depending on nutrition, organ function, and activity
6	Exertion limited	Variable urgency depending on nutrition, organ function, and activity
7	Advanced NYHA lass III symptoms	Transplantation or circulatory support may not be indicated.

cardiogenic shock[28] (**Table 2**). The purpose of this classification was to account for stability versus clinical deterioration and allow for a better understanding of the heterogeneous group, defined as INTERMACS 1.

GUIDELINES

The American College of Cardiology (ACC)/ American Heart Association (AHA) guidelines for HF treatment recommend MCS as a class I

therapy as a BTT.[29] According to the European Society of Cardiology Guidelines,[30] for patients who cannot be stabilized with medical treatment, MCS is suggested to unload the failing ventricle and maintain sufficient end-organ perfusion. Patients in acute cardiogenic shock need to initiate short-term support using extracorporeal, nondurable life support as a bridge to a definitive therapy, which could be medical therapy, durable mechanical support, or heart transplantation. In cases of chronic, refractory

Table 2
Society of Cardiovascular Angiography and Interventions stages of cardiogenic shock

Society of Cardiovascular Angiography Stage and Interventions		Explication
A	At risk	Not experiencing signs or symptoms of cardiogenic shock. Appear well with normal laboratories and physical examination
B	Beginning cardiogenic shock	Relative hypotension and tachycardia without hypoperfusion
C	Classic cardiogenic shock	Hypoperfusion requiring interventions (inotropes/pressors/MCS/ECMO) beyond volume resuscitation. Relative hypotension. Laboratory findings with kidney injury, elevated lactate, brain natriuretic peptide, liver enzymes. Additional invasive hemodynamics with depressed CI
D	Deteriorating/doom	Failure to stabilize despite intense initial efforts and further escalation. At least 30 min elapsed with no resolution of hypotension or hypoperfusion.
E	Extremis	Circulatory collapse in refractory cardiac arrest and ongoing cardiopulmonary resuscitation or supported by simultaneous acute interventions like ECMO

HF, durable mechanical support, or heart transplantation is considered.

SELECTION OF MECHANICAL CIRCULATORY SUPPORT DEVICE

Determining the etiology of refractory failure is the first step when choosing an appropriate device. Next, the clinician identifies if the process is acute or chronic, which chambers are involved (right ventricle [RV], left ventricle [LV], or both), failure of other systems besides cardiac (eg, pulmonary, renal, anhd epatic), and comorbid conditions. A multidisciplinary assessment is utilized to select the best approach.

Currently, there are 3 basic configurations for MCS cannulation for LV support or biventricular support: (1) drainage from right atrium (RA) or inferior vena cava (IVC)/superior vena cava (SVC) and return of blood into the systemic peripheral artery, (2) drainage from LA and return of blood into the systemic peripheral artery (3), and drainage from LV and return of blood to the aorta. For purely RV support, the drainage is from a systemic vein (IVC/SVC) or RA and blood returning into the pulmonary artery (PA) (Fig. 1, Table 3). The devices vary substantially in the amount of added flow they can provide, ranging from 0.5 L/min to 10 L/min. Furthermore, MCS devices provide differential support for the myocardium and the systemic circulation. Although all devices increase the systemic flow and, therefore, perfusion to other organs, their effect on the myocardial tissue differs. Percutaneous LV-aortic (Ao) pumps, such as Impella (Abiomed, Danvers, MA), decrease LV end-diastolic pressure, result in loss of normal isovolumic contraction and relaxation, and decrease myocardial oxygen consumption. On the other hand, devices that drain blood from a systemic vein and return it to the systemic artery tend to increase LV preload and afterload, causing increased myocardial oxygen consumption, pulmonary capillary wedge pressure (PCWP), pulmonary edema, and the risk for LV thrombosis.

ROLE OF PULMONARY ARTERY CATHETERS

Pressure volume loops can offer valuable insight into various MCS devices' direct effects on myocardial mechanics.[31] Pressure-volume loop systems, however, are used mainly for research purposes and are not utilized in clinical practice in most cases. PA catheterization (PAC), on the other hand, is used routinely in clinical practice and serves a valuable role in patient selection for MCS as well as patient monitoring for worsening hemodynamics or signs of recovery. In patients with cardiogenic shock in whom MCS is considered, PACs' routine use should be considered because they provide practical and immediately actionable information in these critically ill patients. PACs allow the determination of RV function and guide the selection of purely LV versus biventricular support. After MCS is initiated, PACs enable the continuous monitoring of cardiac output, and they can help show whether support needs to be escalated before end-organ damage occurs.

Furthermore, PACs continuously monitor RA, PA, and PCWP, and determine myocardial response to circulatory support. Some patients with baseline RV dysfunction show improvement in RA and PA pressures with just LV support; other patients may show progressive right heart dysfunction. This differential impact is based on the degree of support, pulmonary vascular resistance, and underlying RV substrate, among other factors. It is essential to monitor right heart parameters continuously to improve myocardial mechanics and decrease systemic congestion, which can have detrimental effects on kidney and liver function.

In patients supported with an extracorporeal membrane oxygenation (ECMO) device or a similar monitoring configuration, PCWP provides an insight into its impact on LV afterload and preload. If PCWP begins to rise, the patient may require LV venting with another percutaneous or surgical device technique to prevent pulmonary edema and LV thrombosis.

ACUTE HEART FAILURE

Common indications for MCS devices in the acute setting include

1. Post–cardiotomy shock
2. Acute myocarditis
3. Post–myocardial infarction
4. Acute pulmonary embolism (PE)

Post–cardiotomy shock develops after cardiac surgery in patients who cannot be weaned from cardiopulmonary bypass or those who develop low cardiac output in the postoperative period. Various factors determine success after cardiotomy, including timing, support, bleeding control, and adjuvant medical management. In patients with acute myocarditis or cardiogenic shock post–myocardial infarction, the timely initiation of short-term MCS can lead to myocardial recovery.

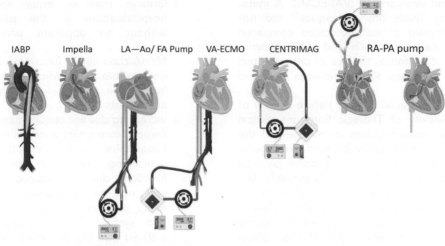

Fig. 1. Schematic depicting configurations for various available temporary MCS devices.

There is a paucity of high-quality randomized controlled data in the field of acute cardiogenic shock due to the acute nature of the disease and difficulties in patient recruitment and randomization. The landmark SHOCK (Should We Emergently Revascularize Occluded Coronaries for Cardiogenic Shock) trial was conducted on refractory cardiogenic shock, and 86% of participants received an intra-aortic balloon pump (IABP) counterpulsation.[32] Mortality was decreased with the use of IABP (72% without IABP vs 57% with IABP; $P = .039$; n = 173) in an unadjusted analysis. After adjusting for catheterization status, however, there was no significant association between mortality and IABP.

The IABP-SHOCK II (Intraaortic Balloon Pump in Cardiogenic Shock II) trial randomly assigned participants planned for early revascularization of acute myocardial infarction complicated with cardiogenic shock to an IABP group or no support group.[33] The IABP-SHOCK II trial did not show an IABP mortality benefit compared with medical therapy at 30 days, 1 year, and 6 years.[33–35] The IABP counterpulsation provides a modest augmentation of the cardiac output of the LV. Because the device requires native ventricular contractility to provide benefit, it may not be sufficient to provide end-organ perfusion in the sickest cohort.

Although the US guidelines still provide IIb (level of evidence [LOE]: B) recommendations for the use of IABP, European guidelines have shifted to class III (LOE: B) recommendations for the use of IABP.[30,36,37] Currently, several other percutaneous MCS devices provide more support than IABP and carry IIb recommendation per current guidelines.[38–40] Recommendations include Impella, LA–femoral artery (FA)

Table 3				
Temporary mechanical circulatory support				
Device		**Indication**		**Support**
IABP	BTR, BTD	LV failure	Acute	0.5–1.0
Impella CP, Impella 2.5, Impella 5.0, Impella 5.5	BTR, BTD	LV failure	Acute	2.5–5.5 L/min
Impella RP	BTR, BTD	RV failure	Acute	2.0–4.0 L/min
LV-Ao pump	BTR, BTD	LV failure	Acute	3.5–5.0 L/min
RA-PA pump	BTR, BTD	RV failure	Acute	Up to 4.5 L/min
VA-ECMO	BTR, BTD, BTC, BTT	RV and/or LV failure	Acute	3–7 L/min
LA-Ao/FA pump	BTR, BTT	RV and/or LV failure	Acute	Up to 10 L/min

bypass, and veno-arterial (VA)-ECMO. A meta-analysis by Thiele and colleagues[41] did not show improved clinical outcomes compared with percutaneous LVADs and IABP. Despite such lack of evidence, the use of percutaneous VADs has increased 30-fold between 2007 and 2012.[42,43]

The 2015 SCAI/ACC/Heart Failure Society of America/Society of Thoracic Surgeons clinical expert consensus provides an overview of the percutaneous MCS alternatives in cardiogenic shock.[44] VA-ECMO, used to support patients with left or biventricular failure, is available, but the optimal unloading mechanisms of the LV still are under investigation. The Survival After Veno-arterial ECMO (SAVE) score can help predict the survival of patients receiving ECMO for refractory cardiogenic shock and, therefore, may aid in patient selection.[45] Extracorporeal life support and ECMO can be employed in acute settings to stabilize hemodynamics, recover end-organ function, and allow a full clinical evaluation for either heart transplant or a more durable MCS device.

Isolated acute RV failure can present in various clinical settings, such as PA hypertension crisis, RV infarct, and acute PE; some patients may require MCS. Acute RV infarct usually accompanies an LV infarct as well, in which case biventricular support may be necessary, but with instances of isolated RV infarct, purely RV support may be sufficient.

CHRONIC HEART FAILURE

Heart transplantation remains a scarce resource with just over 3000 heart transplants performed in the United States annually and fewer than 6000 heart transplants are performed worldwide annually. This limited organ availability and the increasing prevalence of HF patients have led to expanding transplant waiting lists and prolonged waiting times.[8,46] There are, therefore, a growing number of patients needing LVAD support, which has a proved survival benefit for patients on the heart transplant waitlist.[47]

The indications for durable LV assist device implantation include[38,48]

- Patients with greater than or equal to 2 months of severe symptoms despite optimal medical and device therapy and more than 1 of the following:
  - LV ejection fraction less than or equal to 25% and peak Vo2 (volume of oxygen consumption): less than 12 mL/kg/min

  - Greater than or equal to 3 HF hospitalizations in the prior year without an apparent precipitating cause
  - NYHA class IIIb–IV functional limitation despite maximal medical therapy
  - Intolerance to neurohormonal antagonists
  - Increasing diuretic requirements
  - Dependence on intravenous inotropes
  - Progressive end-organ dysfunction (worsening renal and/or hepatic function) due to reduced perfusion and not to inadequate ventricular filling pressure (PCWP $\geq$20 mm Hg and systolic blood pressure [SBP] $\leq$80–90 mm Hg or cardiac index [CI] $\leq$2 L/min/m^2)
  - Absence of severe RV dysfunction.

Durable LVADs can be used as a BTT, recovery, or a destination therapy. When there is appropriate ventricular offloading, LVAD implantation often is associated with a favorable hemodynamic response, improvements in biventricular systolic function, LV end-diastolic volume, PCWP, and pulmonary vascular resistance. Challenges noted with durable MCS include persistent RV failure, aortic insufficiency, gastrointestinal bleeding, anemia, hemolysis, pump thrombosis, stroke, and driveline infection.[49] These complications continue to occur even with the most recent continuous flow magnetically levitated LVADs.[50]

CLINICAL CARE POINTS

Team-based approaches assure that all the providers and collected experience can benefit by streamlining the efforts to improve outcomes.[51,52] One center reported that implementing a standardized team-based approach was associated with a substantial increase in survival in patients with cardiogenic shock (47% to 76.6%).[51] Such impressive results need to be validated in multicenter trials. Nonetheless, this model of care shows a lot of promise in these critically ill patients. In patients presenting with acute PE, a multidisciplinary PE response team (PERT) often is called on for initial risk stratification and the rapid allocation of appropriate resources, such as reperfusion therapies, pulmonary embolectomy, and (in some cases) MCS.[53–55] The authors propose 2 different multidisciplinary team approaches for cardiogenic shock (Fig. 2) and acute PE (Fig. 3) to help the clinicians decide the appropriate mechanical support strategy. The cardiogenic shock team often includes colleagues from critical care cardiology, interventional cardiology, cardiac surgery, advanced HF, and palliative care. PERT members often included vascular medicine, cardiology, pulmonology, hematology, interventional cardiology, and radiology.

CONTROVERSIES AND FUTURE DIRECTIONS

There is a lack of high-quality randomized data for adequately assessing the effects of various MCS options on mortality, complications, and associated morbidities. There is concern about the timing of implantation, device management, patient selection, severity of illness, and variations among institutions.

Ongoing trials include the Danish Cardiogenic Shock Trial (NCT01633502), which is randomizing Impella CP versus conventional circulatory support, and Extra-Corporeal Membrane Oxygenation in the Therapy of Cardiogenic Shock (ECMO-CS), which will randomize patients to VA-ECMO or early conservative therapy. Both studies still are enrolling participants. The National Cardiogenic Shock Initiative (NCT03677180) also will help provide insight into the use of early MCS (Impella) after myocardial infarction and in cardiogenic shock as part of a systemic streamlined algorithm.

The HeartMate PHP (Thoratec Laboratories, Pleasanton, CA) (NCT02279979) is a catheter-based axial flow pump designed to provide partial LV circulatory support currently under investigation.

The ongoing REVERSE (A Prospective Randomised Trial of Early LV Venting Using Impella CP for Recovery in patients with cardiogenic managed with VA ECMO) study (NCT03431467) is aiming to answer the question of LV venting Impella CP while on VA-ECMO support. The lack of LV unloading with VA-ECMO can lead to pulmonary congestion and hamper cardiac recovery, but it may be avoided with a combination of different mechanical options.

For short-term MCS, operators are searching for smaller devices for percutaneous implantation and remote monitoring and control with fewer complications.

New durable support options need to be smaller, more powerful, remotely monitored, transcutaneously chargeable, and with greater hemo-compatibility. There also is an interest in identifying patients who may have the best chance of recovery and investigating therapies that would promote that outcome. The phenomenon of reverse remodeling has been the subject of ongoing research. Cardiac recovery protocols have also emerged in different centers. Other concepts that have become popular recently are door to unloading and cardiac recovery. These concepts are discussed in more detail in subsequent articles. Short-term MCS use with axillary support may aid in the recovery phase of the individuals because early ambulation can help with critical illness and shorter intensive care unit times.

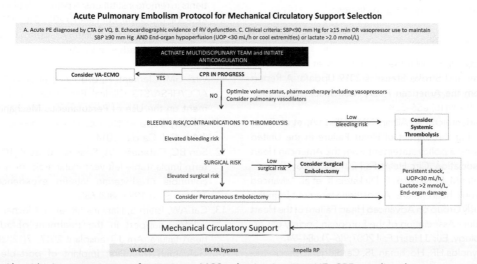

Fig. 2. Algorithmic management of temporary MCS selection in acute HF. CPR, cardiopulmonary resuscitation; CTA, computed tomography angiography; UOP, urine output; VQ, ventilation/perfusion.

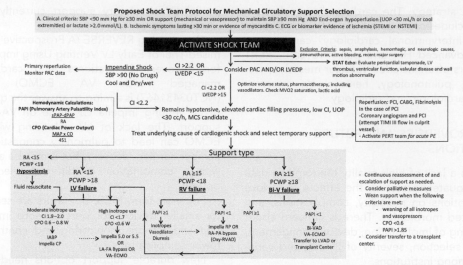

Fig. 3. Algorithmic management of acute massive PE. Bi-V, biventricular; BiVAD, biventricular assist device; CABG, Coronary artery bypass graft; CPO, cardiac power output; CO, cardiac output; dPAP, diastolic pulmonary artery pressure; ECG, electrocardiogram; LVEDP, left ventricular end diastolic pressure; MAP, mean arterial pressure; NSTEMI, non ST elevation myocardial infarction; PAPI, pulmonary artery pulsatility index; PCI, percutaneous coronary intervention; sPAP, systolic pulmonary artery pressure; STAT Echo, stat echocardiogram; STEMI, ST elevation myocardial infarction; TIMI, thrombolysis in myocardial infarction; UOP, urine output.

SUMMARY

MCS provides a variety of options for patients with acute and chronic end-stage HF. There is substantial evidence that short-term and long-term MCS can alleviate symptoms, improve survival rates, and modify disease neurohormonal modulation and reverse remodeling. New technologies are a growing field, and the appropriate selection of therapies in diverse clinical scenarios is of utmost importance.

DISCLOSURE

The authors have nothing to disclose.

REFERENCES

1. Benjamin EJ, Muntner P, Alonso A, et al. Heart Disease and Stroke Statistics-2019 Update: A Report From the American Heart Association. Circulation 2019;139(10):e56–528.

2. Heidenreich PA, Albert NM, Allen LA, et al. Forecasting the Impact of Heart Failure in the United States: a policy statement from the American Heart Association. Circ Heart Fail 2013;6(3):606–19.

3. Metra M, Ponikowski P, Dickstein K, et al. Advanced chronic heart failure: A position statement from the Study Group on Advanced Heart Failure of the Heart Failure Association of the European Society of Cardiology. Eur J Heart Fail 2007;9(6–7):684–94.

4. Reynolds HR, Hochman JS. Cardiogenic shock: current concepts and improving outcomes. Circulation 2008;117(5):686.

5. Babaev A, Frederick PD, Pasta DJ, et al. Trends in management and outcomes of patients with acute myocardial infarction complicated by cardiogenic shock. JAMA 2005;294(4):448.

6. Friedrich EB, Böhm M. Management of end stage heart failure. Heart 2007;93(5):626.

7. Kirklin JK, Naftel DC, Pagani FD, et al. Sixth INTERMACS annual report: A 10,000-patient database. J Heart Lung Transplant 2014;33(6):555.

8. Available at: https://unos.org/data/. Accessed September 1, 2020.

9. Beurtheret S, Mordant P, Paoletti X, et al. Emergency circulatory support in refractory cardiogenic shock patients in remote institutions: A pilot study (the cardiac-RESCUE program). Eur Heart J 2013;34(2):112.

10. Terzi A. Mechanical circulatory support: 60 years of evolving knowledge. Int J Artif Organs 2019;42(5):215–25.

11. Virzì GM, Clementi A, Brocca A, et al. 2015 SCAI/ACC/HFSA/STS Clinical Expert Consensus Statement on the Use of Percutaneous Mechanical Circulatory Support Devices in Cardiovascular Care. J Am Coll Cardiol 2014.

12. Sun BC, Catanese KA, Spanier TB, et al. 100 Long-term implantable left ventricular assist devices: The columbia presbyterian interim experience. Ann Thorac Surg 1999;68(2):688.

13. Cai AW, Islam S, Hankins SR, et al. Mechanical circulatory support in the treatment of advanced heart failure. Am J Transplant 2017;17(12):3020.

14. Goldsmith MF. First implant of portable heart-assist device. JAMA 1991;265(22):2930.

15. Rose EA, Gelijns AC, Moskowitz AJ, et al. Long-term use of a left ventricular assist device for end-stage heart failure. N Engl J Med 2001;345(20):1435.

16. Miller LW, Pagani FD, Russell SD, et al. Use of a continuous-flow device in patients awaiting heart transplantation. N Engl J Med 2007;357(9):885.

17. Wieselthaler GM, O Driscoll G, Jansz P, et al. Initial clinical experience with a novel left ventricular assist device with a magnetically levitated rotor in a multi-institutional trial. J Heart Lung Transplant 2010;29(11):1218.

18. Mehra MR, Uriel N, Naka Y, et al. A fully magnetically levitated left ventricular assist device - Final report. N Engl J Med 2019.

19. Lietz K, Long JW, Kfoury AG, et al. Outcomes of left ventricular assist device implantation as destination therapy in the post-REMATCH era: Implications for patient selection. Circulation 2007;116(5):497.

20. Kalogeropoulos AP, Kelkar A, Weinberger JF, et al. Validation of clinical scores for right ventricular failure prediction after implantation of continuous-flow left ventricular assist devices. J Heart Lung Transplant 2015;34(12):1595.

21. Cowger J, Sundareswaran K, Rogers JG, et al. Predicting survival in patients receiving continuous flow left ventricular assist devices: The Heartmate II risk score. J Am Coll Cardiol 2013;61(3):313.

22. Levy WC, Mozaffarian D, Linker DT, et al. The Seattle Heart Failure Model: Prediction of survival in heart failure. Circulation 2006;113(11):1424.

23. Stevenson LW, Pagani FD, Young JB, et al. INTERMACS profiles of advanced heart failure: the current picture. J Heart Lung Transplant 2009;28(6):535.

24. Aujesky D, Obrosky DS, Stone RA, et al. Derivation and validation of a prognostic model for pulmonary embolism. Am J Respir Crit Care Med 2005;172(8):1041.

25. Matthews JC, Pagani FD, Haft JW, et al. Model for end-stage liver disease score predicts left ventricular assist device operative transfusion requirements, morbidity, and mortality. Circulation 2010;121(2):214.

26. Knaus WA, Draper EA, Wagner DP, et al. APACHE II: A severity of disease classification system. Crit Care Med 1985;13(10):818.

27. Stewart GC, Kittleson MM, Patel PC, et al. INTERMACS (interagency registry for mechanically assisted circulatory support) profiling identifies ambulatory patients at high risk on medical therapy after hospitalizations for heart failure. Circ Heart Fail 2016;9:11.

28. Baran DA, Grines CL, Bailey S, et al. SCAI clinical expert consensus statement on the classification of cardiogenic shock. Catheter Cardiovasc Interv 2019.

29. Hunt SA, Baker DW, Chin MH, et al. ACC/AHA guidelines for the evaluation and management of chronic heart failure in the adult: executive summary. J Heart Lung Transplant 2002;21(2):189–203. https://doi.org/10.1016/s1053-2498(01)00776-8.

30. Ponikowski P, Voors AA, Anker SD, et al. 2016 ESC Guidelines for the diagnosis and treatment of acute and chronic heart failure: The Task Force for the diagnosis and treatment of acute and chronic heart failure of the European Society of Cardiology (ESC) Developed with the special contribution of the Heart Failure Association (HFA) of the ESC. Eur Heart J 2017;37(27):2129.

31. Burkhoff D, Sayer G, Doshi D, et al. Hemodynamics of mechanical circulatory support. J Am Coll Cardiol 2015;66(23):2663–74.

32. Hochman JS, Sleeper LA, Webb JG, et al. Early revascularization in acute myocardial infarction complicated by cardiogenic shock. SHOCK Investigators. Should We Emergently Revascularize Occluded Coronaries for Cardiogenic Shock. N Engl J Med 1999;341(9):625.

33. Thiele H, Zeymer U, Neumann FJ, et al. Intraaortic balloon support for myocardial infarction with cardiogenic shock. N Engl J Med 2012;367(14):1287.

34. Thiele H, Zeymer U, Neumann FJ, et al. Intra-aortic balloon counterpulsation in acute myocardial infarction complicated by cardiogenic shock (IABP-SHOCK II): final 12 month results of a randomised, open-label trial. Lancet 2013;382(9905):1638.

35. Thiele H, Zeymer U, Thelemann N, et al. Intraaortic balloon pump in cardiogenic shock complicating acute myocardial infarction: long-term 6-year outcome of the randomized IABP-SHOCK II trial. Circulation 2018. https://doi.org/10.1161/CIRCULATIONAHA.118.038201. [Epub ahead of print].

36. Ibanez B, James S, Agewall S, et al. 2017 ESC guidelines for the management of acute myocardial infarction in patients presenting with ST-segment elevation: the task force for the management of acute myocardial infarction in patients presenting with ST-segment elevation of the European Society of Cardiology (ESC). Eur Heart J 2018;39(2):119–77.

37. Neumann FJ, Sousa-Uva M, Ahlsson A, et al. 2018 ESC/EACTS guidelines on myocardial revascularization. Eur Heart J 2019;40(2):87–165. https://doi.org/10.1093/eurheartj/ehy394 [published correction appears in Eur Heart J 2019;40(37):3096].

38. Yancy CW, Jessup M, Bozkurt B, et al. 2017 ACC/AHA/HFSA Focused Update of the 2013 ACCF/AHA Guideline for the Management of Heart Failure: A Report of the American College of Cardiology/American Heart Association Task Force on Clinical Practice Guidelines and the

Heart Failure Society of America. J Card Fail 2017;23(8):628.

39. Roffi M, Patrono C, Collet JP, et al. 2015 ESC guidelines for the management of acute coronary syndromes in patients presenting without persistent ST-segment elevation: task force for the management of acute coronary syndromes in patients presenting without persistent ST-Segment Elevation of the European Society of Cardiology (ESC). Eur Heart J 2016;37(3):267–315. https://doi.org/10.1093/eurheartj/ehv320.

40. Sjauw KD, Engström AE, Vis MM, et al. A systematic review and meta-analysis of intra-aortic balloon pump therapy in ST-elevation myocardial infarction: Should we change the guidelines? Eur Heart J 2009;30(4):459.

41. Thiele H, Jobs A, Ouweneel DM, et al. Percutaneous short-term active mechanical support devices in cardiogenic shock: a systematic review and collaborative meta-analysis of randomized trials. Eur Heart J 2017;38(47):3523–31. https://doi.org/10.1093/eurheartj/ehx363.

42. Khera R, Cram P, Lu X, et al. Trends in the use of percutaneous ventricular assist devices: Analysis of National Inpatient Sample data, 2007 through 2012. JAMA Intern Med 2015;175(6):941.

43. Sandhu A, McCoy LA, Negi SI, et al. Use of mechanical circulatory support in patients undergoing percutaneous coronary intervention: insights from the National Cardiovascular Data Registry. Circulation 2015;132(13):1243.

44. Rihal CS, Naidu SS, Givertz MM, et al. 2015 SCAI/ACC/HFSA/STS Clinical Expert Consensus Statement on the Use of Percutaneous Mechanical Circulatory Support Devices in Cardiovascular Care (Endorsed by the American Heart Association, the Cardiological Society of India, and Sociedad Latino Americana de Cardiología Intervencionista; Affirmation of Value by the Canadian Association of Interventional Cardiology-Association Canadienne de Cardiologie d'intervention). Catheter Cardiovasc Interv 2015;85(7):1112.

45. Amin F, Lombardi J, Alhussein M, et al. Predicting survival after VA-ECMO for refractory cardiogenic shock: validating the SAVE score. CJC Open 2020;3(1): 71–81. https://doi.org/10.1016/j.cjco.2020.09.011.

46. Taylor DO, Stehlik J, Edwards LB, et al. Registry of the International Society for Heart and Lung Transplantation: Twenty-sixth Official Adult Heart

Transplant Report-2009. J Heart Lung Transplant 2009;28(10):1007.

47. Trivedi JR, Cheng A, Singh R, et al. Survival on the heart transplant waiting list: Impact of continuous flow left ventricular assist device as bridge to transplant. Ann Thorac Surg 2014;98(3):830.

48. Crespo-Leiro MG, Metra M, Lund LH, et al. Advanced heart failure: a position statement of the Heart Failure Association of the European Society of Cardiology. Eur J Heart Fail 2018;20(11): 1505–35. https://doi.org/10.1002/ejhf.1236.

49. Kirklin JK, Naftel DC, Pagani FD, et al. Seventh INTERMACS annual report: 15,000 patients and counting. J Heart Lung Transplant 2015;34(12): 1495.

50. Kormos RL, Cowger J, Pagani FD, et al. The Society of Thoracic Surgeons Intermacs database annual report: evolving indications, outcomes, and scientific partnerships. J Heart Lung Transplant 2019; 38(2):114–26. https://doi.org/10.1016/j.healun.2018.11.013.

51. Tehrani BN, Truesdell AG, Sherwood MW, et al. Standardized team-based care for cardiogenic shock. J Am Coll Cardiol 2019;73(13):1659–69. https://doi.org/10.1016/j.jacc.2018.12.084 [published correction appears in J Am Coll Cardiol 2019;74(3):481].

52. Rivera-Lebron B, McDaniel M, Ahrar K, et al. Diagnosis, treatment and follow up of acute pulmonary embolism: consensus practice from the PERT consortium. Clin Appl Thromb Hemost 2019;25. https://doi.org/10.1177/1076029619853037. 1076029619853037.

53. Jen WY, Kristanto W, Teo L, et al. Assessing the impact of a pulmonary embolism response team and treatment protocol on patients presenting with acute pulmonary embolism. Heart Lung Circ 2020;29(3):345–53. https://doi.org/10.1016/j.hlc.2019.02.190.

54. Chaudhury P, Gadre SK, Schneider E, et al. Impact of multidisciplinary pulmonary embolism response team availability on management and outcomes. Am J Cardiol 2019;124(9):1465–9. https://doi.org/10.1016/j.amjcard.2019.07.043.

55. Myc LA, Solanki JN, Barros AJ, et al. Adoption of a dedicated multidisciplinary team is associated with improved survival in acute pulmonary embolism. Respir Res 2020;21(1):159. https://doi.org/10.1186/s12931-020-01422-z.

Vascular Access for Large Bore Access

Stephen McHugh, MD[a], Ali Noory, MD[a], Suraj Mishra, MD[a],
Catherine Vanchiere, MD[a], Vladimir Lakhter, DO[b],*

KEYWORDS

- Vascular access • Large bore • Ultrasound guidance • Micropuncture needle • Hemostasis

---

KEY POINTS

- Using a micropuncture needle and ultrasound guidance is key to obtaining safe femoral artery access.
- Both anatomic landmarks and fluoroscopy are needed to ensure optimal needle entry into common femoral artery at the level of mid-femoral head.
- Antegrade perfusion of the distal leg may be needed to reduce the risk of limb ischemia during large bore vascular access.
- Ability to obtain adequate hemostasis after removal of a large bore sheath is critical to reducing the rate of vascular complications.

INTRODUCTION

Since the time of the first successful human cardiac catheterization in 1929,[1] there has been a tremendous amount of innovation and progress in the realm of coronary angiography and intervention. As the complexity of interventional procedures has evolved, so has the need for safe percutaneous vascular access. Although most coronary interventions can be performed using a 6 French sheath, large bore vascular access is required for patients undergoing transcatheter aortic valve replacement (TAVR), Impella placement and initiation of venoarterial extracorporeal membrane oxygenation (V-A ECMO). In the present article, the authors review some of the important features involved in large bore vascular access including vascular anatomy, technical aspects of femoral artery access, potential complications, anatomic challenges, hemostasis, and alternative access.

ARTERIAL ANATOMY
Radial Artery

Radial artery (RA) is 1 of the 2 arteries that arises from the bifurcation of the brachial artery at the level of the antecubital fossa (along with the ulnar artery). The ulnar and radial arteries have communications within the palm via the deep and superficial palmar arches. The Allen test is typically used to test the patency of the palmar arch.[2]

In recent years, the RA has become the artery of choice for performing coronary angiography and percutaneous coronary intervention. The average size of the RA is approximately 2 to 3 mm, and it can therefore accommodate a 5 French (outer diameter – 2.49 mm) or a 6 French (outer diameter – 2.77 mm) sheath.[3] Although 7 French access can be possible with the use of 6/7 French Slender sheaths (Terumo, Somerset, New Jersey) or using a sheathless guide (Terumo), the size of the RA is generally prohibitive for placement of larger bore access.

---

[a] Department of Medicine, Temple University Hospital, Lewis Katz School of Medicine, 3401 North Broad Street, Philadelphia, PA 19140, USA; [b] Division of Cardiovascular Diseases, Department of Medicine, Temple University Hospital, Lewis Katz School of Medicine, 3401 North Broad Street (9PP), Philadelphia, PA 19140, USA
* Corresponding author.
E-mail address: Vladimir.lakhter@tuhs.temple.edu

Intervent Cardiol Clin 10 (2021) 157–167
https://doi.org/10.1016/j.iccl.2020.12.004

Iliofemoral Arteries

The infrarenal abdominal aorta typically bifurcates at the level of the fourth lumbar vertebrae into the right and left common iliac arteries (average diameter between 9 and 10 mm).[4] Common iliac artery bifurcates into the internal iliac artery (which provides the arterial supply to the pelvis) and the external iliac artery (EIA). The EIA courses within the retroperitoneal space up to the point of the inguinal ligament, at which point the artery courses anteriorly and is renamed a common femoral artery (CFA – average diameter of 6 mm).[5] The CFA is bound superiorly by the inferior epigastric artery and inferiorly by its bifurcation point into the profunda femoris and superficial femoral arteries (SFAs – average diameter of 5 mm).

The CFA is a commonly used location for large bore vascular access. Unless significant stenosis is present, the average CFA size should allow for placement of an arterial sheath as large as 16 to 18 French. As will be described in later sections, great care should be taken to access the artery at a location where successful hemostasis can be obtained. Furthermore, the large bore sheath may be occlusive to the artery and may thus compromise distal blood flow. Several techniques have been developed to allow for perfusion of the distal extremity, while the large bore access remains in place and will be detailed in a later section.

Axillary Artery

Large bore access using the axillary artery (AA) has recently emerged as a safe alternative to the CFA approach. In a retrospective analysis of 110 computed tomography (CT) scans at a single institution, the mean diameter of the AA was measured to be 6.38 mm on the right and 6.52 mm on the left; this is comparable to the average sized CFA and therefore compatible with large bore sheath placement. Furthermore, the AA had lower rates of stenosis and calcification compared with the iliofemoral arteries.[6]

The AA is divided into 3 segments:

The proximal or first section lies between the lateral margin of the first rib and medial border of the pectoralis minor muscle.

The second segment lies deep to the pectoralis minor muscle.

The third and more distal segment lies between the lateral pectoralis minor muscle and inferior border of the teres major muscle.

In order to reduce the risk of a pneumothorax or injury to the brachial plexus, the AA should be accessed between the second and third portions. Angiographically, the ideal access location should be lateral to the thoracoacromial artery and medial to the circumflex humeral arteries.[7]

Transcaval Anatomy

Transcaval access (which will be described in more detail later in the article) is another alternative location for large bore sheath placement. A large bore sheath is initially inserted into the common femoral vein and advanced to the level of the infrarenal inferior vena cava. At this point, the sheath is intentionally crossed over through the IVC wall and into the infrarenal abdominal aorta, thereby bypassing the iliofemoral arteries all together. An ideal anatomic location for transcaval access is at the level of the infrarenal abdominal aorta that appears the least calcified. Identifying this location requires meticulous preprocedural planning, ideally with CT angiography of abdomen and pelvis.

FEMORAL ARTERY ACCESS

The CFA is among the most frequently used sites for vascular access. Although the use of transradial access for coronary angiography and percutaneous coronary intervention has increased over the recent years,[8] CFA access remains necessary for many diagnostic and therapeutic interventions, especially if large bore access is required. The femoral artery is less prone to spasm compared with the RA and is comparably less problematic when repeated access is required.[9] It is also the preferred access site for technically complex procedures such as transcatheter aortic valve replacement (TAVR), endovascular aortic aneurysm repair, and percutaneous mechanical support device insertion such as Impella CP and V-A ECMO.[10,11]

The key to successful placement of a large bore arterial sheath is to first ensure that the CFA is accessed carefully and safely. This section will explore the important aspects of successful CFA sheath placement.

Technical Considerations for Common Femoral Artery Access
Anatomy

As noted earlier, the CFA is the continuation of the EIA, which emerges at the midway point of the inguinal ligament and runs parallel to the medial aspect of the femoral head. At its origin, the CFA is bordered by the femoral vein medially and the anterior crural nerve laterally. It is covered anteriorly by fascia extending from the transverse abdominis and iliac muscles. Together, these structures form the femoral sheath.[12] The CFA then passes through the sheath to bifurcate into the SFA and profunda femoris artery branches.[5]

The ideal location for arterial sheath insertion within the CFA is halfway between the inferior epigastric artery (which arises from the EIA right above the level of the inguinal ligament) and CFA bifurcation. In order to identify the proper location for needle entry, various traditional methods have to be used in tandem. These include palpatory identification of the inguinal crease, the bony landmarks, and the point of maximal CFA impulse. Additional use of nonpalpatory techniques such as fluoroscopy, ultrasound guidance, use of micropuncture needles, and femoral angiography have also shown to improve success rates.

Inguinal crease
The inguinal crease has been an often used landmark that is assumed to identify the anatomic course of the inguinal ligament. Nevertheless, studies have shown that there can be a significant variation in distance between the crease and the ligament, ranging from 0 to 11 cm (with an average distance of 6.5 cm).[13] In addition, other studies have found that the CFA bifurcation occurs proximal to the crease in over 75% of patients.[14] This is especially true in obese individuals in whom the location of the crease is displaced caudally by the panus. Therefore, the use of the inguinal crease may be an unreliable guide for CFA puncture, which can lead to a low stick.

Bony landmarks
Being that the true course of the inguinal ligament is approximated by an imaginary line between the bony protrusion of the anterior superior iliac spine (ASIS) superiorly and the pubic symphysis inferiorly, identification of these bony landmarks can be useful at the time of CFA access.[5,15,16] After noting the location of these bony landmarks with a marker, several techniques have been described for accessing CFA relative to the position of the inguinal ligament. One technique aims for needle puncture at the midpoint of a line drawn between the ASIS and the pubic symphysis.[17] Alternatively, another technique suggests to puncture perpendicular and 2.5 cm caudal to this line.[18] It is important to note the palpation of the ASIS and the pubic symphysis is not possible in every patient, as these bony protrusions can be obscured in presence of obesity, residual hematoma, or scarred tissue from previous intervention.[12]

Maximal femoral impulse
Locating the femoral artery's point of maximal arterial impulse has been suggested to be a more reliable means of guiding access to the CFA than the use of the inguinal crease. The strongest palpable sensation of the femoral pulse was shown to be located over the CFA in over 92% of limbs where a strong pulse was palpable.[14] Nevertheless, this technique is rendered difficult in patients with significant vascular disease who may have poorly palpable or absent femoral pulsations.

Fluoroscopy
Although performing a complete anatomic evaluation using the palpatory methods outlined previously is important for obtaining successful CFA access, additional assessment is often needed.

Fluoroscopic identification of the center of the femoral head can be a significant aid at the time of arterial access. Studies have shown that CFA is located over the medial half of the femoral head 97% of the time, and in most cases the CFA bifurcation is located approximately 3.5 cm caudal to the midpoint of the femoral head.[19] Therefore, the skin level over the midfemoral head should be identified by placing a hemostat on top of the skin while performing fluoroscopy. A marker line can then be traced onto the skin over the top of the hemostat and be used as a target for arteriotomy (it should be noted that the needle has to enter the skin below this line; the distance from the line depends on the patient's body habitus and the angle of needle entry).

Aside from allowing the identification of the femoral head, fluoroscopy can allow for direct fluoroscopy-guided puncture. This can prove to be particularly useful in morbidly obese patients in whom anatomic landmarks cannot be palpated and in patients with weak or impalpable pulses.[20] In this technique, the femoral head is visualized fluoroscopically and placed into the center view. The needle can then be aimed toward the CFA based on its expected location over the medial part of the femoral head. The technique has a greater chance for success in cases of severe CFA calcification (in which case the CFA outline is seen on fluoroscopy). Alternatively, target for CFA access can be identified by performing a contrast injection from the contralateral up-and-over CFA access or by placing a wire in an up-and-over fashion that can serve as the target for needle entry.

Ultrasound guidance for vascular access
Ultrasound guidance at the time of CFA access is an invaluable tool that allows for direct visualization of the CFA and its bifurcation. Ultrasound

use can decrease the chance of low arterial puncture, reduce the risk of pseudoaneurysm formation, and help avoid inadvertent entry into the common femoral vein.[21]

The Femoral Arterial Access with Ultrasound Trial (FAUST) was the largest study to examine the use of ultrasound for guiding CFA access.[22] FAUST was a prospective, multicenter trial that randomized 1004 patients to either fluoroscopic or ultrasound-guided CFA access. The primary endpoint, which evaluated the rate of successful femoral arterial cannulation, was similar in both groups. However, ultrasound guidance was found to increase the odds of CFA sheath placement among patients with high CFA bifurcation. Ultrasound use also reduced the number of attempts needed to obtain access, reduced the risk of venipuncture, and decreased the time needed for sheath insertion. There was also a significant reduction in access site complications, namely in preventing the development of hematomas greater than 5 cm in size. Importantly, there was no difference in the rate of high sticks. Subsequent meta-analysis showed that ultrasound guidance was associated with a 49% reduction in overall complications compared with traditional CFA access techniques.[23]

Micropuncture

The use of a micropuncture needle (21-gauge) offers a smaller arteriotomy size (56% size reduction) at the time of access compared to the traditional 18-gauge Cook needle (Cook, Bloomington, Indiana). This is especially useful in patients who are obese and/or fully anticoagulated.[24] After obtaining a brisk bleed-back from the end of the micropuncture needle (the flow may not be pulsatile because of the small needle gauge), a micropuncture wire is inserted through the needle and directed toward the ipsilateral iliac artery. At this point, it is important to perform fluoroscopy to ensure that the micropuncture wire is following the expected anatomic course of the external and common iliac arteries. At times, the wire may enter the circumflex iliac artery; in this case the wire will appear to deviate toward the lateral aspect of the pelvis rather than course toward the aortic bifurcation. The wire should be pulled be and redirected in order to avoid perforation of the distal circumflex iliac artery.

Fluoroscopy will also identify the location of the radiopaque distal tip of the micropuncture needle in relation to the femoral head (Fig. 1). In the event of unintended needle entry into either a low or high part of the vessel (ie, below or above the level of the femoral head), the

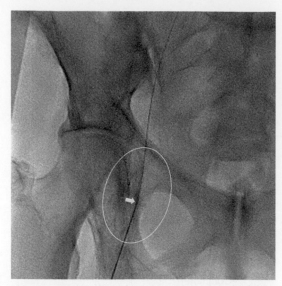

Fig. 1. Fluoroscopic image of micropuncture needle entry at the level of the lower third of the femoral head. The yellow arrow designates the transition point between the needle tip and the micropuncture wire.

needle can be removed and quick hemostasis obtained after several minutes of manual compression. Although the studies examining the role of micropuncture compared with standard needle access have not shown significant differences in complications rates, the studies are nonrandomized and therefore difficult to interpret.[24–27]

Putting it all together

Femoral artery access should ideally be obtained using a combination of the previously described techniques (such as ultrasound with fluoroscopy and the use of micropuncture needle) to ensure reliable sheath placement into the mid-CFA segment and to reduce the risk of complications.[28] After attempting to locate the bony anatomic landmarks and determining the approximate location of the inguinal ligament, the middle portion of the femoral head is identified using fluoroscopy. A radiopaque object such as a hemostat can next be used to mark the femoral head's surface position on the skin. Then, targeted ultrasound guidance is used to identify the CFA and its bifurcation point in relation to the marked skin surface over the mid-femoral head.

After administering local anesthesia, targeted puncture and CFA access are performed under directed ultrasonographic guidance. Once successful arterial sheath placement is achieved, angiography of the CFA should be performed using ipsilateral oblique angulation (30°–40°) +/− digital subtraction (Fig. 2). Angiography will help identify the exact point of sheath entry

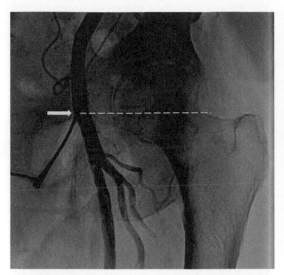

Fig. 2. Common femoral artery angiography performed through the sidearm of the femoral arterial sheath. The dashed line demonstrates the point of sheath at the level of lower third of the femoral head.

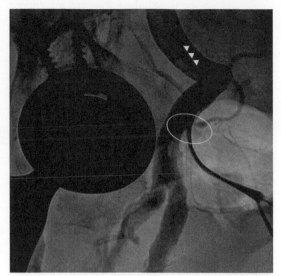

Fig. 3. Common femoral artery sheath angiography showing extreme tortuosity of the distal external iliac artery. Yellow arrow heads designate the 0.035 inch wire that is kept inside the sheath during contrast injection in order to reduce the risk of hydraulic vessel dissection within the tortuous segment. The yellow circle shows the sheath entry into at the level of the mid femoral head.

relative to the location of the CFA bifurcation and the takeoff of the inferior epigastric artery. Knowing the location of sheath entry is important for understanding whether a closure device can be used to achieve hemostasis at the end of the case. Additionally, it will help define the vessel size, anatomy/tortuosity, and calcification. It is important to keep the 0.035 inch wire inside the sheath while performing femoral sheath angiography; the wire helps to keep the tip of the sheath off the arterial wall and can therefore reduce the risk of hydraulic vessel dissection (**Fig. 3**).

For cases in which large bore CFA access is planned, performing a nonselective aorto-iliac angiography can further define the size and morphology of the common and external iliac arteries. Aortoiliac angiography can be performed by advancing a catheter with side holes (such as a Pigtail or Omniflush) into the infrarenal abdominal aorta (L2 vertebrae) and performing a contrast injection (eg, 30 mL of contrast at 20 mL/s, 1000 PSI, 0.0 rise time) under digital subtraction (3 frames/s). After selecting the laterality for large bore access, Perclose sutures can be placed as part of a preclose technique (described in detail in a later section). The arteriotomy site is then serially dilated, and a large bore sheath is advanced.

Ipsilateral Antegrade Limb Perfusion
A unique consideration for patients requiring large bore CFA access is the possibility of compromised arterial supply distal to sheath insertion. This is a particular concern for patients

with concomitant peripheral artery disease (PAD) involving the lower extremities; in these patients, there is a real risk of limb ischemia.[29,30] Therefore, insertion of an antegrade perfusion catheter may be needed to avoid limb compromise. Several antegrade perfusion techniques have been described and are discussed in detail in another section of this series.

COMPLICATIONS

Vascular complications occur in 1% to 9% of all patients undergoing vascular access placement. Developing a vascular complication results in prolonged hospital stay, higher health care costs, and increased rates of mortality (specifically in patients undergoing percutaneous intervention for acute myocardial infarction).[31–33] Risk factors include female sex, older age, being overweight or underweight, uncontrolled hypertension, the use of large bore arterial sheaths, prolonged sheath duration, and concomitant use of anticoagulants.[9] Although there are many possible vascular complications, this article will highlight hematoma formation, retroperitoneal bleeding, arteriovenous fistula, and pseudoaneurysm formation.

Hematoma Formation
Bleeding is the most common complication of transfemoral access. It can manifest as minor bleeding at the puncture site, ecchymoses, and

hematoma formation; these can generally be controlled with limited manual pressure. In more severe cases, prolonged manual pressure or application of a hemostatic device may be required. Some patients may require reversal of anticoagulation therapy and volume/blood product resuscitation. If patients become hemodynamically unstable,[34] further evaluation may be required to rule out retroperitoneal bleeding or pseudoaneurysm rupture.

Retroperitoneal Bleeding

Retroperitoneal (RP) bleeding represents a significant complication associated with femoral arterial access and occurs in less than 3% of all patients undergoing CFA access.[35] The greatest predictor of RP bleeding is a high arterial stick, especially if it is superior to the takeoff of the inferior epigastric artery. Additional risk factors include low body weight, female sex, left femoral puncture, larger sheath size, and concomitant use of glycoprotein IIb/IIIa inhibitors.[36,37] In patients suspected of having an RP bleed, an urgent CT scan of the abdomen/pelvis without contrast should be performed. Although most cases can be managed conservatively, a subset of patients will require additional endovascular or surgical intervention.

Arteriovenous Fistula

The incidence of arteriovenous (AV) fistula formation following CFA access is less than 1%. AV fistulas are abnormal communications between the femoral artery and vein at the site of sheath insertion; the blood flow is directed from the high-pressure artery into the low-pressure vein and results in left-to-right shunting. Risk factors for AV fistula formation include multiple attempts at femoral access, low puncture site (the profunda femoris vein lies close to the SFA), large sheath sizes, female sex, and ineffective manual compression.[38] Although AV fistulas are rarely symptomatic, in severe cases patients can develop high-output heart failure, lower extremity edema, and arterial steal syndrome. Most small fistulas resolve spontaneously and only require observation with serial ultrasound examinations. Larger AV fistulas and those that are symptomatic should be undergo treatment with ultrasound-guided manual compression, surgical ligation, endovascular stent graft insertion, or coil embolization.

PSEUDOANEURYSM

The incidence of iatrogenic femoral pseudoaneurysm (PSA) formation varies between 1%

and 3%. PSA most commonly results from insufficient hemostasis of the arteriotomy with resultant bleeding and formation of a pseudo-wall that stops the blood from continuous extravasation into the surrounding tissue. Risk factors include large sheath size, ineffective manual compression, and low puncture sites (below the level of CFA bifurcation).

On examination, patients are most often found to have a pulsatile groin mass and an audible bruit. Diagnosis is made using an arterial doppler ultrasound. For PSAs under 2 cm, observation and serial doppler evaluation are recommended. Treatment for larger PSAs consists of ultrasound-guided compression, thrombin injection, covered stent placement, and surgical repair.[37]

ANATOMIC CHALLENGES

Although the femoral artery is the most commonly used access for large bore vascular sheath placement, there are several anatomic considerations that present unique challenges. These include excessive tortuosity and heavy calcification.

TORTUOSITY

Severe arterial tortuosity of the common and external iliac arteries can make it difficult to advance an arterial sheath of any size, let alone a large bore sheath. Success in overcoming tortuosity depends on several key factors. First, the need for stiff 0.035 inch wires that allow for straightening of the tortuous segments; these wires include the Supracore (Abbott, Chicago, Illinois), Amplatz Super Stiff (Boston Scientific, Marlborough, Massachusetts), Amplatz Extra Stiff (Cook, Bloomington, Indiana) and Lunderquist wires (Cook) Upfront advancement of a stiff wire is unlikely to be successful at first, and therefore the tortuous segment should initially be crossed with a soft wire such as a Wholey (Medtronic, Minneapolis, Minnesota), Bentson (Cook), or a Soft angled Glidewire (Terumo, Somerset, New Jersey). A straight catheter (such a Glidecath) can then be advanced into the descending aorta, and an exchange of a soft wire for a stiff wire can take place. The second factor is the importance of placing a long sheath (25-35 cm long) whose proximal segment will terminate in the infrarenal aorta rather than within the tortuous iliac artery segment. Finally, it is important to recognize that even while using a stiff wire, the stiff sheath dilator may not easily track up the vessel. If resistance is encountered upon sheath advancement, further attempts to overcome the resistance may result in significant vessel injury such as perforation or dissection. In these cases, using balloon-assisted tracking or an inch-worming technique can be helpful.[39]

CALCIFICATION

Presence of arterial calcification can be another major challenge to obtaining successful large bore arterial access. Severity of calcification can be assessed using different imaging modalities such as fluoroscopy, CT, and peripheral intravascular ultrasound (IVUS). Of these, IVUS[40] can provide the most detailed information regarding the extent of calcification; this information in turn can be useful in understanding whether adjunctive therapies may be needed at the time of arterial access.

HEMOSTASIS

Successful hemostasis after removal of the large bore arterial sheath is a crucial final step of any procedure. The options for hemostasis include manual compression, percutaneous closure, and primary surgical repair. Manual compression, which is used routinely for smaller caliber sheaths (such as 5 and 6 French) may not be a great option for larger sheaths (ie, Impella and TAVR sheaths), especially in obese patients. Instead, percutaneous closure (using any of the commercially available vascular closure devices [VCDs]) may achieve a more rapid and definitive hemostasis. In situations where percutaneous closure is not possible (ie, heavily calcified or diseased CFA) primary surgical repair may be the best hemostatic option.

Percutaneous Hemostasis
Although there are many available VCDs, this discussion will focus on Perclose and Manta closure devices.

Suture-mediated hemostasis
The Perclose Proglide device (Abbott, Chicago, Illinois) is a suture-mediated system designed to achieve hemostasis via percutaneous delivery of a single suture adjacent to the arteriotomy site. For any sheath size larger than 8 French, 2 Percloses are recommended to be deployed in a preclose fashion. In a preclose technique,[41] the Percloses are deployed at 10 p.m. and 2 p.m. positions relative to the arteriotomy site prior to large bore sheath insertion. Once the sheath is removed, the sutures are tightened using the knot pusher, which is included in the Perclose kit. Of note, some operators do not use 2

Percloses and instead elect to use a single Perclose in combination with a 6 or 8 French Angioseal (Terumo, Somerset, New Jersey).[42]

An alternative approach to achieving Perclose suture-mediated hemostasis is to use the postclose technique in which Percloses are deployed after sheath removal. This is especially useful in situations where large bore arterial access was obtained without initial placement of Perclose sutures (ie, emergency Impella placement). The challenge of the postclose technique is that the Perclose sutures may not adequately capture the vessel wall after large bore sheath removal, because the arteriotomy defect is significantly bigger then the diameter of the Proglide. One way to increase the likelihood of successful hemostasis[43] is to replace the large bore sheath with 2 smaller sheaths (eg, replacing a 14 French sheath with 2 7 French sheaths). One of the smaller sheaths is then removed and the first Perclose deployed while keeping the second smaller sheath in place. Having the second smaller sheath across the arteriotomy may serve to bias the suture entry into the arterial wall rather than through the posterior vessel wall. If the first Perclose is successfully deployed, the second small sheath is then removed and the second Perclose delivered. This technique can be assisted by inflating a balloon (sized 1:1 with the vessel) in the ipsilateral external iliac artery using an up-and-over approach from the contralateral CFA (dry close). Low pressure balloon inflation is performed after the large bore access is removed and serves to reduce the amount of bleeding during sheath exchange and Perclose delivery.

Complications related to suture-mediated hemostasis are rare.[44] Nevertheless, early recognition is important, as it can allow for rapid intervention to be instituted. The most commonly encountered Perclose-related complications are stenosis, dissection, and occlusion of the arterial site. These can be easily recognized by performing a lower extremity angiogram after tightening of the sutures; angiography is frequently performed either via the contralateral common femoral artery (up-and-over) or radial artery (**Fig. 4**).

MANTA
More recently, a new product called MANTA (Teleflex, Morrisville, New Jersey) was US Food and Drug Administration approved for biomechanical vascular closure of sheaths ranging from 10 to 20 French (12-25 French outer diameter). The device is similar in action the Angioseal closure device and works by deploying a

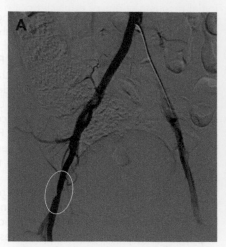 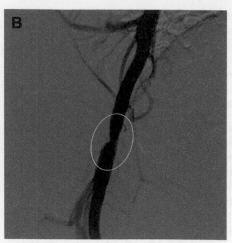

Fig. 4. (*A*) Iliofemoral digital subtraction angiography of the right lower extremity after Perclose performed using an up-and-over injection. (*B*) Close-up of the common femoral artery reveals a patent vessel with a focal area of mild stenosis related to the Perclose sutures (*yellow circle*).

bioabsorbable plug on the inner aspect of the arteriotomy site. There is also a small nonabsorbable radiopaque marker that is left on the external surface of the arteriotomy. The IFU for MANTA warns against using this device in patients with severe CFA calcification, diseased CFA with diameter less than <5 mm (14 French device) or less than 6 mm (18 French device), or in patients with severe PAD.

The safety and efficacy of the device were studied in 263 patients as part of the prospective, multicenter SAFE MANTA IDE[45] clinical trial. Technical success rate was 97.7% with mean time from deployment to hemostasis of 65 seconds. There was a 5.3% rate of major complications (defined as vascular injury requiring surgical repair/stent-graft, bleeding requiring transfusion, lower extremity ischemia requiring surgical repair/additional percutaneous intervention, nerve injury [permanent or requiring surgical repair], and infection requiring intavenous antibiotics and/or extended hospitalization) and a 4.2% rate of VARC-2 major vascular complications.

ALTERNATIVE ACCESS

Although a CFA approach is the preferred site for large bore sheath placement, in some patients this access point is not feasible. Failure to obtain successful CFA access is predominantly related to anatomic factors such as excessive tortuosity, heavy calcification, or advanced atherosclerotic involvement of the iliofemoral arteries. In these situations, alternative access for large bore sheath placement may be required.

This section will briefly highlight the axillary and transcaval approaches.

Axillary Artery Access

As noted earlier, the AA is similar in size to the CFA; however, it is less likely to be stenosed or calcified. There are 2 main approaches to accessing the axillary artery: needle entry through the axilla[46] and needle entry through the inferior border of the clavicle.[47] Although needle access through the axilla allows the needle to travel through a smaller amount of soft tissue and potentially allow for easier hemostasis, there is a higher potential risk of brachial plexus injury. Alternatively, needle insertion below the clavicle largely avoids the brachial plexus; however, this makes hemostasis challenging because of the inability to achieve good manual compression over the arteriotomy.

The general approach to hemostasis for AA access that is obtained with the infraclavicular needle entry is by using the preclose technique. However, unlike the preclose technique for CFA access in which manual pressure can be applied to the access site during Proglide exchanges, similar manual pressure cannot be applied effectively to AA site. Instead, low pressure balloon inflation within the ipsilateral subclavian artery can be used to control the bleeding. The balloon is positioned into the subclavian artery over on 0.018 inch wire that is inserted through a small bore (5 or 6 French) CFA access. Controlled balloon inflations are also used at the end of the procedure once it is time to remove the large bore sheath.

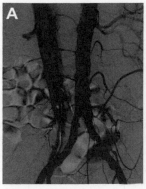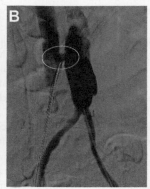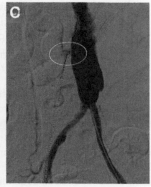

Fig. 5. (A) Simultaneous inferior vena cava gram and aortoiliac angiogram performed prior to transcaval access. (B) Yellow circle illustrates a significant left-to-right shunt that occurs immediately after removal of the large bore transcaval access. (C) Almost complete resolution of the left-to-right shunt following successful placement of a PDA occluder.

Transcaval Access

Large bore transcaval access involves bypassing the iliofemoral arteries in favor of the iliofemoral veins and creating a sheath-mediated channel between the abdominal aorta and the inferior vena cava. As noted previously, this requires meticulous preprocedural imaging with CT angiography. Because the presence of aortic calcium presents a significant impediment for transcaval access, anatomic planning is used to identify the location within the abdominal aorta that is most conducive and calcium free for a transcaval approach. The access spot should be paired to the vertebral body in a similar axial cut of the CTA to allow easy identification in the catherization laboratory. At the time of the procedure, this anatomic target should be confirmed with simultaneous IVC venography and abdominal aortic angiography (Fig. 5A).

As with AA access, achieving successful hemostasis after transcaval access is of critical importance. Hemostasis is generally achieved by placement of a closure device (such as a PDA occluder; Fig. 5A, B) across the IVC and abdominal aortic defects.[7,48]

Clinics care points

- Use of ultrasound guidance at the time of vascular access improves successful CFA access and reduces the number of attempts.
- Safe femoral access requires the combination of multiple techniques including careful assessment of anatomic landmarks, ultrasound guidance and use of micropuncture.
- Although access-related vascular complications are rare, they require immediate attention to reduce morbidity.

- Alternative vascular access site (such as axillary and trascaval) are feasible and can be done safely following careful preprocedural planning.

DISCLOSURE

The authors have nothing to disclose.

REFERENCES

1. Mueller RL, Sanborn TA. The history of interventional cardiology: cardiac catheterization, angioplasty, and related interventions. Am Heart J 1995;129(1):146–72.
2. Greenwood MJ, Della-Siega AJ, Fretz EB, et al. Vascular communications of the hand in patients being considered for transradial coronary angiography: is the Allen's test accurate? J Am Coll Cardiol 2005;46(11):2013–7.
3. Ashraf T, Panhwar Z, Habib S, et al. Size of radial and ulnar artery in local population. J Pak Med Assoc 2010;60(10):817–9.
4. Pederson OM, Aslaksen A, Vik-Mo H. Ultrasound measurement of the luminal diameter of the abdominal aorta and iliac arteries in patients without vascular disease. J Vasc Surg 1993;17(3):596–601.
5. Spector KS, Lawson WE. Optimizing safe femoral access during cardiac catheterization. Catheter Cardiovasc Interv 2001;53(2):209–12.
6. Tayal R, Iftikhar H, LeSar B, et al. CT angiography analysis of axillary artery diameter versus common femoral artery diameter: implication for axillary approach for transcatheter aortic valve replacement in patients with hostile aortoiliac segment and advanced lung disease. Int J Vasc Med 2016; 2016:3610705.
7. Cheney AE, McCabe JM. Alternative percutaneous access for large bore devices. Circ Cardiovasc Interv 2019;12(6):e007707.

8. Feldman DN, Swaminathan RV, Kaltenbach LA, et al. Adoption of radial access and comparison of outcomes to femoral access in percutaneous coronary intervention: an updated report from the National Cardiovascular Data Registry (2007-2012). Circulation 2013;127:2295–306.

9. Irani F, Kumar S, Colyer W. Common femoral artery access techniques: a review. J Cardiovasc Med (Hagerstown) 2009;10(7):517–22.

10. Webb JG, Wood DA. Current status of transcatheter aortic valve replacement. J Am Coll Cardiol 2012;60:483–92.

11. Werdan K, Gielen S, Ebelt H, et al. Mechanical circulatory support in cardiogenic shock. Eur Heart J 2014;35:156–67.

12. Van Den Berg J. Optimal technique for common femoral artery access. Endovascular Today 2013;1. Available at: https://evtoday.com/articles/2013-jan/optimal-technique-for-common-femoral-artery-access?c4src=archive:feed. Accessed August 10, 2020.

13. Lechner G, Jantsch H, Waneck R, et al. The relationship between the common femoral artery, the inguinal crease, and the inguinal ligament: a guide to accurate angiographic puncture. Cardiovasc Intervent Radiol 1988;11:165–9.

14. Grier D, Hartnell G. Percutaneous femoral artery puncture: practice and anatomy. Br J Radiol 1990; 63:602–4.

15. Sherev DA, Shaw RE, Brent BN. Angiographic predictors of femoral access site complications: implication for planned percutaneous coronary intervention. Catheter Cardiovasc Interv 2005;65: 196–202.

16. Schnyder G, Sawhney N, Whisenant B, et al. Common femoral artery anatomy is influenced by demographics and comorbidity: implications for cardiac and peripheral invasive studies. Catheter Cardiovasc Interv 2001;53:289–95.

17. Lumley JSP, Craven JL, Aitken JT. Essential anatomy. 4th edition. Edinburgh (Scotland): Churchill Livingstone; 1987. p. 229.

18. McKears D, Owens R. Surface anatomy for radiographers. Bristol (England): Wright; 1979. p. 96–7.

19. Dotter CT, Rosch J, Robinson M. Fluoroscopic guidance in femoral artery puncture. Radiology 1978;127:266–7.

20. Jacobi JA, Schussler JM, Johnson KB. Routine femoral head fluoroscopy to reduce complications in coronary catheterization. Proc (Bayl Univ Med Cent) 2009;22:7–8.

21. Gabriel M, Pawlaczyk K, Waliszewski K, et al. Location of femoral artery puncture site and the risk of postcatheterization pseudoaneurysm formation. Int J Cardiol 2007;120:167–71.

22. Seto AH, Abu-Fadel MS, Sparling JM, et al. Real-time ultrasound guidance facilitates femoral arterial access and reduces vascular complications: FAUST (Femoral Arterial Access with Ultrasound Trial). J Am Coll Cardiol Intv 2010;3:751–8.

23. Sobolev M, Slovut DP, Lee Chang A, et al. Ultrasound-guided catheterization of the femoral artery: a systematic review and metaanalysis of randomized controlled trials. J Invasive Cardiol 2015;27:318–23.

24. Baker NC, Ansel GM, Rao SV, et al. The choice of arterial access for percutaneous coronary intervention and its impact on outcome: an expert opinion perspective. Am Heart J 2015;170:13–22.

25. Ambrose JA, Lardizabal J, Mouanoutoua M, et al. Femoral micropuncture or routine introducer study (FEMORIS). Cardiology 2014;129:39–43.

26. Mignatti A, Friedmann P, Slovut DP. Targeting the safe zone: a quality improvement project to reduce vascular access complications. Catheter Cardiovasc Interv 2018;91(1):27–32.

27. Ben-Dor I, Maluenda G, Mahmoudi M, et al. A novel, minimally invasive access technique versus standard 18-gauge needle set for femoral access. Catheter Cardiovasc Interv 2012;79:1180–5.

28. Sandoval Y, Burke MN, Lobo AS, et al. Contemporary arterial access in the cardiac catheterization laboratory. JACC Cardiovasc Interv 2017;10:2233–41.

29. Gerhard-Herman MD, Gornik HL, Barrett C, et al. 2016 AHA/ACC guideline on the management of patients with lower extremity peripheral artery disease: executive summary: a report of the American College of Cardiology/American Heart Association Task Force on Clinical Practice Guidelines. Circulation 2017;135:e686–725.

30. Kurra V, Schoenhagen P, Roselli EE, et al. Prevalence of significant peripheral artery disease in patients evaluated for percutaneous aortic valve insertion: preprocedural assessment with multidetector computed tomography. J Thorac Cardiovasc Surg 2009;137:1258–64.

31. Yatskar L, Selzer F, Feit F, et al. Access site hematoma requiring blood transfusion predicts mortality in patients undergoing percutaneous coronary intervention: data from the National Heart, Lung, and Blood Institute Dynamic Registry Catheter. Cardiovasc Interv 2007;69:961–6.

32. Kinnaird TD, Stabile E, Mintz GS, et al. Incidence, predictors, and prognostic implications of bleeding and blood transfusion following percutaneous coronary interventions. Am J Cardiol 2003;92::930–5.

33. Romaguera R, Wakabayashi K, Laynez-Carnicero A, et al. Association between bleeding severity and long-term mortality in patients experiencing vascular complications after percutaneous coronary intervention. Am J Cardiol 2012;109:75–81.

34. Bhatty S, Cooke R, Shetty R, et al. Femoral vascular access-site complications in the cardiac catheterization laboratory: diagnosis and management. Interv Cardiol 2011;3(4):503–14.

35. Femoral arterial access and complications. The Cardiology Advisor. Available at: https://www.the-cardiologyadvisor.com/home/decision-support-in-medicine/cardiology/femoral-arterial-access-and-complications/. Accessed August 10, 2020.

36. Ellis SG, Bhatt D, Kapadia S, et al. Correlates and outcomes of retroperitoneal hemorrhage complicating percutaneous coronary intervention. Catheter Cardiovasc Interv 2006;67(4):541–5.

37. Kronzon I. Diagnosis and treatment of iatrogenic femoral artery pseudoaneurysm: a review. J Am Soc Echocardiogr 1997;10:236–45.

38. Kelm M, Perings SM, Jax T, et al. A prospective study on incidence and risk factors of arteriovenous fistulae following transfemoral cardiac catheterization. J Am Coll Cardiol 2012;40(2):291–7.

39. Grenon SM, Reilly LM, Ramaiah VG. Technical endovascular highlights for crossing the difficult aortic bifurcation. J Vasc Surg 2011;54(3):893–6.

40. Shammas NW, Radaideh Q, Shammas WJ, et al. The role of precise imaging with intravascular ultrasound in coronary and peripheral interventions. Vasc Health Risk Manag 2019;15:283–90.

41. Lata K, Kaki A, Grines C, et al. Pre-close technique of percutaneous closure for delayed hemostasis of large-bore femoral sheaths. J Interv Cardiol 2018; 31(4):504–10.

42. Amponsah MK, Tayal R, Khakwani Z, et al. Safety and efficacy of a novel "hybrid closure" technique in large-bore arteriotomies. Int J Angiol 2017; 26(2):116–20.

43. Thawabi M, Cohen M, Wasty N. Post-close technique for arteriotomy hemostasis after Impella removal. J Invasive Cardiol 2019;31(6):E159.

44. Vinayakumar D, Kayakkal S, Rajasekharan S, et al. 24h and 30 day outcome of Perclose Proglide suture mediated vascular closure device: an Indian experience. Indian Heart J Jan-Feb 2017;69(1):37–42.

45. Wood DA, Krajcer Z, Sathananthan J, et al. Pivotal clinical study to evaluate the safety and effectiveness of the MANTA percutaneous vascular closure device. Circ Cardiovasc Interv 2019;12(7):e007258.

46. Hallak A, Wei L, Berzingi C, et al. Percutaneous axillary access for large-bore arteriotomy: A step-by-step guide. J Card Surg 2018;33(5):270–3.

47. Mathur M, Hira RS, Smith BM, et al. Fully percutaneous technique for transaxillary implantation of the Impella CP. JACC Cardiovasc Interv 2016; 9(11):1196–8.

48. Lederman RJ, Greenbaum AB, Rogers T, et al. Anatomic suitability for transcaval access based on computed tomography. JACC Cardiovasc Interv 2017;10(1):1–10.

Mechanical Circulatory Support in Acute Myocardial Infarction and Cardiogenic Shock

Alejandro Lemor, MD, MSc[a], Lina Ya'qoub, MD[b],
Mir B. Basir, DO, FSCAI[a,c,*]

KEYWORDS

- Acute myocardial infarction • Cardiogenic shock • Mechanical circulatory support
- Intra-aortic balloon pump • Extracorporeal membrane oxygenation • TandemHeart • Impella

KEY POINTS

- Acute myocardial infarction complicated by cardiogenic shock is a deadly condition associated with significant morbidity and mortality.
- Despite 20 years of medical advancements, early revascularization remains the sole therapy proven to improve outcomes.
- Mechanical circulatory support devices provide a physiologically plausible mechanism of improving outcomes by offering hemodynamic stability for revascularization and improving end-organ perfusion. Results from well-powered randomized controlled trials, however, are not yet available.
- Randomized controlled trials have been difficult to conduct in this patient population; until such trials are performed, implementing shock teams and protocols has been associated with improved outcomes in observational studies and may be considered.
- Technological advancements will lead to continued development of more mobile, smaller-caliber, and more powerful mechanical circulatory support devices. Understanding the mechanisms of action and physiologic effects of these devices, therefore, is critically important.

INTRODUCTION

Acute myocardial infarction (AMI) can result in diastolic dysfunction and an increase in left ventricular end-diastolic pressure. If not treated promptly, AMI can progress to systolic dysfunction and decreasing stroke volume, which can lead to cardiogenic shock (CS). CS is a low-output state resulting in decreased systemic and coronary perfusion. Decreased systemic perfusion results in end-organ injury, whereas decreased coronary perfusion results in further ischemia, leading to a vicious cascade that ultimately can lead to death. The cascade of events results in a complex neurohumoral cascade referred to as the systemic inflammatory response syndrome. The goals for treating AMI and CS (AMICS), therefore, are to relieve ischemia and improve perfusion to end organs.[1]

AMICS is a deadly condition associated with significant morbidity and mortality. Patients presenting with AMICS who do not receive invasive

A. Lemor and L. Ya'qoub contributed equally to this article.
[a] Henry Ford Health Care System, 2799 West Grand Blvd, K-2 Cath Lab, Detroit, MI 48202, USA; [b] Louisiana State University, One University Place, Shreveport, LA 71115, USA; [c] Henry Ford Hospital, 2799 West Grand Boulevard (K-2 Cath Lab), Detroit, MI 48202, USA
* Corresponding author. STEMI, Acute Mechanical Circulatory Support, Henry Ford Hospital, 2799 West Grand Boulevard (K-2 Cath Lab), Detroit, MI 48202.
E-mail address: Mbasir1@hfhs.org

therapies have less than 20% survival.[2] The Should We Emergently Revascularize Occluded Coronaries for Cardiogenic Shock (SHOCK) trial demonstrated improved survival in patients presenting with AMICS treated with early mechanical revascularization.[3] Unfortunately, further revascularization does not lead to further improvements in short-term survival, as was demonstrated in the CULPRIT-SHOCK trial.[4] In the past 2 decades, there has been little advancement made to improving outcomes further. This is of great concern because the prevalence of AMICS is growing in the aging population.[5] Patients frequently present with more comorbidities and are more likely to experience cardiac arrest and CS.[5]

Given the high mortality associated with AMICS despite revascularization, clinicians have looked to other forms of therapies in the hope of improving outcomes. Technological advancements have resulted in an increased availability of temporary mechanical circulatory support (MCS) devices, which can improve systemic and coronary perfusion. These devices are reviewed herein.

INTRA-AORTIC BALLOON PUMP

Intra-aortic balloon pump (IABP) counterpulsation is the oldest and most common form of MCS.[6–8] Since its inception in 1967, several observational studies have suggested improved survival with the use of IABP in patients with AMICS[9–21] (Table 1). IABPs have been demonstrated to improve systemic hemodynamics and improve coronary perfusion, are easy to use, and are inexpensive. Until recently, there was 1 alternative device, venoarterial (VA)–extracorporeal membrane oxygenation (ECMO), which was more invasive, associated with more complications, and utilized primarily in select tertiary care centers. Therefore, the use of IABPs was questioned infrequently for decades.

Randomized controlled trials (RCTs), however, failed to show survival benefit[22–26] (Table 2). In the Thrombolysis and Counterpulsation to Improve Cardiogenic Shock (TACTICS) trial, 57 patients with AMICS were randomized after thrombolytic therapy to 48 hours of IABP therapy or optimal medical therapy. The investigators found no significant difference in 6-month mortality between the 2 groups.[22] Prondzinsky and colleagues[24] randomized 45 patients with AMICS after percutaneous coronary intervention (PCI) to IABP therapy or optimal medical therapy. They found no difference in Acute Physiology and Chronic Health Evaluation II scores,

interleukin-6 levels, and cardiac index (CI) between the groups. In-hospital mortality also was similar between the groups (38.6% vs 28.6%, respectively).[24] The largest trial conducted evaluating the efficacy of IABP in AMICS was the IABP-SHOCK II trial; 300 patients were randomized to IABP and 298 patients to the control group. There was no difference in outcomes, including secondary endpoints, such as time to hemodynamic stabilization, length of stay in the intensive care unit, serum lactate levels, dose and duration of catecholamine therapy, renal function, major bleeding, peripheral ischemic complications, and stroke.[25,26]

Furthermore, numerous meta-analyses have investigated the role of routine IABP in AMICS.[27–29] The largest analysis was performed by Ahmad and colleagues,[27] who analyzed patients presenting with AMI from 12 RCTs, including 2123 patients, and 15 observational studies, including 15,530 patients. They found no difference in 30-day mortality in patients with AMI who received IABP, regardless of the presence (odds ratio [OR] 0.94; 95% CI, 0.69–1.28) or absence (OR 0.98; 95% CI, 0.57–1.69) of CS.[28] As a result of these randomized trials and meta-analyses, the European guidelines downgraded IABP use in AMICS from a previous class I to a class III recommendation,[30] whereas the US guidelines downgraded IABP use to a class II recommendation.[31]

This review focuses on patients with AMICS. Patients who present with CS from decompensated heart failure CS, however, differ in their response to IABPs. Malick and colleagues[32] have demonstrated that patients with decompensated heart failure CS had a 5-fold greater cardiac output augmentation with IABP compared with patients with AMICS.

VENOARTERIAL–EXTRACORPOREAL MEMBRANE OXYGENATION

VA-ECMO uses a centrifugal pump and a membrane oxygenator, to provide flows of up to 3 L/min to 7 L/min. There are few retrospective observational studies evaluating the use of ECMO in AMICS (Table 3). These studies demonstrate a survival rate ranging from 47% to 60.9% in patients who have a mean age of 54 years to 60 years.[33,34] In 2010, Sheu and colleagues[35] studied 115 patients with AMICS from 1993 to 2002 without ECMO support and compared them with 219 patients with AMICS from 2002 to 2009 with ECMO support. The 30-day mortality for patients with ECMO was lower than the non-ECMO cohort (30.1% vs

Table 1
Summary of observational studies of intra-aortic balloon pump in acute myocardial infarction and cardiogenic shock

Author, Year Published	Number of Patients	Population	Outcomes
Moulopoulos et al,[9] 1986	N = 52 34 IABP	AMICS	10/34 patients survived longer than a month. 15 patients in whom IABP could not be placed, none survived
Bengtson et al,[10] 1992	N = 200 99 IABP	AMICS	In-hospital mortality 53% Patency of infarct-related vessel was a predictor of survival. No difference between IABP and no IABP arms
Waksman et al,[11] 1993	N = 85 20 IABP	AMICS	In-hospital and 1-y survival was significantly higher in the IABP arm (46% and 38% vs 19% and 10%, respectively; $P<.001$).
Stomel et al,[12] 1994	N = 64 13 thrombolytics 29 IABP 22 thrombolytics + IABP	AMICS	Survival improved in thrombolytics + IABP group compared with thrombolytics or IABP alone (68% vs 23% or 28%, respectively; $P = .0049$).
Anderson et al,[13] 1997	N = 310 68 IABP	AMICS	Despite more adverse events and moderate bleeding, the IABP cohort showed a trend toward lower 30-d and 1-y mortality rates.
Kovack et al,[14] 1997	N = 46 patients 27 IABP	AMICS who received thrombolytics	Patients in the IABP arm had significantly higher hospital survival (93% vs 37%, respectively; $P = .0002$).
Brodie et al,[15] 1999	N = 1490	AMI with and without CS	Pre-PCI IABP was associated with lower cardiac events in CS (n = 119) (14.5% vs 35.1%, respectively; $P = .009$), in CHF or low ejection fraction (n = 119) (0% vs 14.6%, respectively; $P = .10$), and in high-risk patients (n = 238) (11.5% vs 21.9%, respectively; $P = .05$).
Kumbasar et al,[16] 1999	N = 45 25 IABP	Anterior AMI who received thrombolytics	IABP had significantly higher rates of thrombolysis in myocardial infarction grade 3 flow (n: 11%; 44% vs n: 1%, respectively; 5%; $P<.05$). There was a

(continued on next page)

Author, Year Published	Number of Patients	Population	Outcomes
			trend toward a lower in-hospital mortality in the IABP group (n: 0 [0%] vs n: 3; [15%]; $P = .08$).
Sanborn et al,[17] 2000	N = 856 279 IABP, 160 IABP + thrombolytics 132 thrombolytics only	AMICS	Thrombolytic group had a lower in-hospital mortality compared with no-thrombolytics (54% vs 64%, respectively; $P = .005$). The IABP group had a lower in-hospital mortality compared with no-IABP (50% vs 72%, respectively; $P<.0001$).
Barron et al,[18] 2001	N = 23,180 7268 IABP	AMICS	IABP was associated with significantly lower mortality in the thrombolytic group (67% vs 49%, respectively) but not in PCI group (45% vs 47%, respectively).
Zeymer et al,[19] 2011	N = 653 163 IABP	AMICS	In-hospital mortality, with and without IABP, was 56.9% and 36.1%, respectively. In the multivariate analysis the use of IABP was not associated with improved survival (OR 1.47; 95% CI, 0.97–2.21; $P = .07$).
Sjauw et al,[20] 2012	N = 292 199 IABP	STEMI with CS treated with PCI	30-d mortality in IABP vs no-IABP was 47% vs 28%, respectively; OR 1.67 (95% CI, 1.16–2.39), no difference after propensity stratification 3-d mortality in pre-PCI IABP vs post-PCI was 64% vs 40%, respectively; OR of 1.56 (95% CI, 1.18–2.08), no difference after propensity stratification
Zeymer et al,[21] 2013	N = 1913 487 IABP	AMICS	In-hospital mortality with and without IABP was 43.5% and 37.4% respectively. In multivariate analysis, IABP was associated with increased mortality (OR 1.45; 95% CI, 1.15–1.84).

Table 2
Summary of randomized clinical trials of intra-aortic balloon pump in acute myocardial infarction and cardiogenic shock

Author, Year Published	Number of Patients	Population	Outcomes
Ohman et al,[22] 2005	57 patients	AMICS who received thrombolytics	No difference in 6-mo mortality (34% for IABP + thrombolytics vs 43% for thrombolytics alone [n = 27]; adjusted P = .23)
Prondzinsky et al,[24] 2010	45 patients	AMICS status post-PCI	No difference in in-hospital mortality, Acute Physiology and Chronic Health Evaluation II scores, interleukin-6 levels, and CI at 4 d.
Thiele et al,[25] 2012	598 patients	AMICS	No difference in 30-d mortality, the time to hemodynamic stabilization, the length of stay in the intensive care unit, serum lactate levels, the dose and duration of catecholamine therapy, renal function, major bleeding, peripheral ischemic complications, and stroke
Thiele et al,[26] 2018	591 patients	AMICS	No difference in 6-y mortality, recurrent myocardial infarction, stroke, repeat revascularization, or rehospitalization for cardiac reasons

41.7%, respectively; P = .034). A subgroup analysis of patients in profound CS found a significant difference in mortality between groups (39.1% in ECMO vs 72% in non-ECMO; P = .008); however, in patients without profound shock, there was no significant difference in 30-day mortality between the groups (26.1% vs 21.9%, respectively; P = .39). Esper and colleagues[36] studied 18 patients who underwent VA-ECMO in the catheterization laboratory for AMICS and found an in-hospital survival rate of 67% and 6-month survival of 55%. More than one-third of patients had an IABP placed and were on vasopressors or inotropes. Similarly, Negi and colleagues[37] studied 15 patients with AMICS (one-third presenting with cardiac arrest) and showed a 47% survival rate. More than 90% of patients were on 1 to 2 inotropes at the time of ECMO, 60% had an IABP, and the vascular complication rate was greater than 50%. Lastly, a recent observational study by Vallabhajosyula and colleagues[38] using the National Inpatient Sample database evaluated 2962 patients in a period of 14 years and demonstrated a survival

rate of 40.8%. There was a significant trend to improved survival over time and 12% of patients were bridged to LV assist device (LVAD) or heart transplantation.[38]

There are no RCTs to date evaluating the use of ECMO in AMICS. Two European studies, EURO SHOCK and ECLS-SHOCK, currently are enrolling patients. EURO-SHOCK will randomize 428 patients to ECMO or standard therapy and will evaluate 30-day mortality as the primary outcome; their expected study completion date is February 2024.[39] Similarly, ECLS-SHOCK will enroll 420 patients with AMICS undergoing revascularization and randomize to ECMO or medical therapy alone. The primary outcome is 30-day mortality and the estimated study completion date is August 2023.[40]

TandemHeart

TandemHeart (LivaNova, London, UK) used a percutaneous centrifugal pump to provide flows up to 3 L/min to 5 L/min using cannulas similar to VA-ECMO. There are few studies assessing the

Table 3
Major observational studies of venoarterial–extracorporeal membrane oxygenation in acute myocardial infarction and cardiogenic shock

Author/Trial (Year)	Sample Size	Observational Studies Device (s)	Results	Notes
Esper et al,[36] 2015	18	VA-ECMO	67% survival rate, very high bleeding rates (>90%)	Single-center experience, peripheral ECMO, average length of ECMO was 3.2 d ± 2.5 d
Negi et al,[37] 2016	15	VA-ECMO	47% survival rates, 53% vascular complication rates	Small sample, single center, 33% with cardiac arrest, 60% with STEMI
Sheu et al,[35] 2010	219	VA-ECMO	60.9% survival in ECMO vs 28% survival in the non-ECMO cohort	All patients prior to ECMO had a IABP and were on dobutamine
Takayama et al, 2013	90	VA-ECMO	49% survival.	Combined AMI and CHF patients in shock; 23 patients underwent permanent LVAD and 9 heart transplantation.
Vallabhajosyula et al, 2019	2962	ECMO	40.8% survival	Survival improved from 0% in 2000– to 54.9% in 2014. Potential bias due to administrative database. Multicenter, large sample study

hemodynamic and clinical outcomes of Tandem-Heart in patients with AMICS (Table 4). Kar and colleagues[41] studied 80 patients with AMICS and found that TandemHeart led to a rapid improvement several hemodynamic measures, including CI, systolic blood pressure, urine output, and lactic acid levels. The mortality rates were 40.2% and 45.3% at 30 days and 6 months, respectively, for AMICS patients. Smith and colleagues[42] analyzed 56 patients, 16 (29%) of whom had AMICS, and found improved hemodynamics with the use of TandemHeart. They also found that survival was significantly influenced by the indication of the TandemHeart (23.8% in bridge to recovery vs 51% in bridge to LVAD or surgery [P = .04]), and patients who did not receive definitive therapy had poor outcomes (13.8% survived to hospital discharge). Further observational data are being collected in the TandemHeart Experiences and MEthods (THEME Registry); an ongoing

multicenter study (ClinicalTrials.gov Identifier: NCT02326402).

Two underpowered RCTs have been conducted with the use of TandemHeart. Thiele and colleagues[43] randomized 20 patients to IABP and 21 patients to TandemHeart. They found cardiac power index and other hemodynamics measures improved more effectively with TandemHeart; however, complications, including severe bleeding and limb ischemia, were more frequent. The investigators also found no difference in 30-day mortality between groups; however, the study was underpowered to detect these differences.[43] Burkhoff and colleagues[44] randomized 33 patients with AMICS to treatment with IABP or TandemHeart. They similarly found improved hemodynamics with higher CI and lower pulmonary capillary wedge pressure with the use of TandemHeart; however, there was no difference in 30-day mortality between the groups.[44]

Table 4
Major studies of TandemHeart in acute myocardial infarction and cardiogenic shock

Study, Publication Year	Number of Patients	Study Type	Outcomes
Thiele et al, 2005	41	RCT: IABP vs TandemHeart	No difference in 30-d mortality. TandemHeart led to improvement in hemodynamics but was associated with more complications, including bleeding and limb ischemia.
Burkhoff et al,[44] 2006	33	RCT: IABP vs TandemHeart	No difference in 30-d mortality. TandemHeart led to improvement in hemodynamics.
Kar et al,[41] 2011	117 total, 80 with AMI, 37 with NICM	Observational: TandemHeart in refractory shock	30-d and 6-mo mortality rates were 40.2% and 45.3%, respectively, in AMI, vs 32% and 35%, respectively, in NICM. TandemHeart led to improvement in hemodynamics.
Smith et al,[42] 2018	56 total, 16 (29%) AMI	Observational, CS due to advanced HF and AMI	Survival was significantly influenced by indication (23.8% in bridge to recovery vs 51% in bridge to LVAD or surgery; $P = .04$). TandemHeart led to significant improvements in CI and PCWP.
Schwartz et al, 2012	76, 19 received TandemHeart, 58% AMI	Observational	30-d mortality 63%

Abbreviations: NICM, nonischemic cardiomyopathy; PCWP, pulmonary capillary wedge pressure.

IMPELLA

Impella (Abiomed, Danvers, Massachusetts) is continuous nonpulsatile micro-axial pump that has an inlet area that aspirates blood from the left ventricle and ejects it through the outlet into the ascending aorta, at a rate up to 5.5 L/min. Observational studies assessing the use of Impella in CS have compared it with either medical therapy, IABP, or ECMO (Table 5). The Impella-EUROSHOCK registry was an observational-single arm study that evaluated 120 patients with AMICS supported with an Impella 2.5. The feasibility study demonstrated a 64% 30-day mortality; however, it showed feasibility of device placement and improvement in lactate levels.[45] Karatolios and colleagues[46] compared Impella to medical therapy in 90 patients with cardiac arrest (27 patients were treated with Impella) and demonstrated 65% survival in the Impella cohort compared with 20% in the medical therapy cohort. Schrage and colleagues[47] matched patients from the IABP-SHOCK II trial to patients supported with an Impella device in Europe. They demonstrated

no significant difference in 30-day all-cause mortality (48.5% vs 46.4%, respectively; $P = .64$) but did show higher rates of severe bleeding and vascular complications in the Impella group. The main limitation of this study was that the degree of CS was not taken into account when matching patients. Lemor and colleagues[48] analyzed AMICS patients from the National Inpatient Sample from 2015 to 2017 who underwent PCI and had either Impella or ECMO support. Propensity-matched analysis showed significantly lower mortality in the Impella cohort (26.7% vs 43.3%, respectively; $P = .02$) as well as lower ischemic stroke and vascular complication rates. This study, however, also was limited by the inability to match patients according to the degree of shock. Loehn and colleagues[49] showed improved survival with the use of Impella before PCI (50% pre-PCI Impella vs 23.1% post-PCI Impella). Helgestad and colleagues[50] demonstrated lower 30-day mortality in patients receiving Impella compared with a matched control group that underwent IABP placement (40% vs 77.5%, respectively; P log rank <0.001).

Table 5
Summary of randomized controlled trials and observational studies for Impella

Randomized Controlled Trials

Author/Trial (Year)	Sample Size	Comparison	Results	Notes
ISAR-SHOCK[51] (2008)	12 vs 13	Impella 2.5 vs IABP	Similar 30-d mortality in both groups (46% for both)	Improved CI with Impella device
IMPRESS[52] (2017)	24 vs 24	Impella CP vs IABP	Similar 30-d (46% vs 50%, respectively; P = .92) and 6 mo mortality (50% for both; P = .9)	>90% of patients with cardiac arrest prior device placement

Observational studies

Author/Trial (Year)	Sample Size	Device (s)	Results	Notes
INOVA[60] (2019)	82	IABP, Impella, ECMO	30-survival was 63.4% for all patients (62/82 supported with Impella)	A multidisciplinary team–based approach can improve outcomes.
NCSI[59] (2019)	171	Impella CP	72% survival with best practices (early RHC, MCS, and PCI)	Lactate <4 and cardiac power output >0.6 are good predictors of survival. Multicenter study
Utah Cardiac Recovery Shock Team[64] (2019)	123	IABP, Impella, ECMO	54.5% survival (for the entire cohort—IABP, Impella, ECMO)	33.3% of patients supported with Impella. AMICS in 61%
Schrage et al,[49] 2019	237 matched patients from IABP-SHOCK trial	Impella CP vs IABP	No difference in survival (48.5% vs 46.4%, respectively; P = .64)	Selection bias and unable to compare degree of shock between patients
EUROSHOCK[45] (2013)	120	Impella 2.5	64% 30-d mortality	Impella is feasible and reduced lactate levels
Karatolios et al,[46] 2018	90	Impella CP vs medical therapy	65% survival in Impella cohort vs 20% with medical therapy (27/90 with Impella support)	All patients had cardiac arrest. Single-center study

Study	Comparison	N	Results	Comments
Lemor et al,[48] 2020	Impella CP vs ECMO	5730 vs 560 (450 propensity matched)	Propensity matched: in-hospital mortality rates were 26.7% vs 43.3%, respectively.	Potential bias due to administrative database. Multicenter, large sample study
Loehn et al,[49] 2020	Impella CP	73	50% survival for Impella Pre-PCI vs 23.1% for Impella post-PCI	More patients in the Impella post-PCI group had cardiac arrest, although younger patients in the Impella pre-PCI group with higher percentage of left main disease.
Helgestad et al,[50] 2020	Impella CP vs IABP	903 (279 with MCS)	Lower 30-d mortality compared with matched control group (40% vs 77.5%, respectively; P log rank <0.001).	Matched cohort included 40 patients in each group.

Abbreviation: RHC, right heart cath.

Two underpowered RCTs have been conducted evaluating Impella in AMICS. Both compared Impella versus IABP in a small sample of patients. The ISAR-SHOCK trial randomized 25 patients to either Impella 2.5 or IABP and demonstrated safety and feasibility to use Impella 2.5 in AMICS. Patients treated with Impella had similar 30-day mortality when compared with IABP (46%); however, Impella did provide better hemodynamic support.[51] The IMPella versus IABP Reduces mortality in STEMI patients treated with primary PCI in Severe cardiogenic SHOCK (IMPRESS) trial was a randomized, prospective, open-label, multicenter trial that enrolled 48 patients with AMICS and randomized patients to an Impella CP or IABP.[52] The investigators aimed to enroll more than 100 patients but the trial was prematurely stopped due to poor enrollment. Overall, the results showed similar mortality rates for both cohorts (46% for Impella and 50% for IABP; $P = .9$).

RIGHT VENTRICULAR FAILURE

Acute right coronary artery occlusion proximal to the right ventricular (RV) branches, or less commonly left circumflex artery occlusion, often results in RV ischemia. RV ischemia can lead to depressed RV systolic function decreasing transpulmonary flow and left ventricular filling. This can result in diminished preload and cardiac output. The severity of the hemodynamic compromise in patients with RV failure is related to the extent of RV ischemia, left ventricular function, and ventricular interdependence.[53] Patients with RV dysfunction are prone to bradyarrhythmias, which can further decrease cardiac output. Hemodynamic compromise from RV failure, therefore, should be treated first with volume resuscitation, restoration of physiologic rhythm or pacing, and inotropic agents. Patients with persistent RV failure can be considered for RV MCS devices.

In patients with left ventricular dysfunction, increased left ventricular pressures and pulmonary venous pressures lead to increased RV afterload, which further decreases RV output. Lala and colleagues[54] analyzed patients from the SHOCK trial, which recruited primarily patients with left ventricular failure and found that the prevalence of RV failure (ie, biventricular failure) was 38%. They defined RV failure using hemodynamic parameters: central venous pressure greater than 10 mm Hg, central venous pressure/pulmonary capillary wedge pressure greater than 0.63, pulmonary artery pulsatility index less than 2, and RV stroke work index less

than 450 g*m/m². Using similar definitions, Basir and colleagues demonstrated similar findings in the National Cardiogenic Shock Initiative (NCSI) and identified these patients as having increased mortality compared with those with isolated left ventricular failure.

VA-ECMO is a powerful RV assist device (RVAD), and, in the setting of concomitant left sided failure, may be the preferred modality of MCS, because it provides biventricular support. Unfortunately, data on its use specifically for RV failure in the setting of AMICS are limited.

The Impella RP is a percutaneous microaxial pump designed to support the RV. There are few data demonstrating the impact of Impella RP on outcomes in patients with RV dysfunction (Table 6). Cheung and colleagues[55] studied 18 patients, 39% of whom had AMI and found that Impella RP led to improvements in hemodynamic measures and reported a 30-day survival rate of 72% and a 1-year survival rate of 50%. The RECOVER RIGHT study included 30 patients with RV failure refractory to medical therapy. The investigators found that patients had improvement in hemodynamics with the use of an Impella RP. Overall, 73.3% of patients survived to 30 days.[56]

TandemHeart–RVADs (TH-RVADs) use an extracorporeal centrifugal flow pump and 2 venous cannulas to deliver blood from the right atrium (RA) to the main PA via bilateral femoral venous cannulation. A 21F inflow cannula is placed in the RA and a second 21F outflow cannula is inserted into the main PA. Usually, the outflow cannula is placed in the main PA via the right femoral vein, and the inflow cannula is placed in the RA via the left femoral vein. If the distance from femoral vein to fifth intercostal space exceeds 58 cm or femoral access cannot be used, the internal jugular venous access can be utilized. There also is a ProtekDuo (LivaNova, London, UK) dual-lumen cannula, which can be placed in the right internal jugular vein. It contains 2 lumens within one 29F or 31F cannula, taking blood from RA to the extracorporeal pump then delivering it to the PA. There are few data on the use of TH-RVAD on outcomes (see Table 5). Kapur and colleagues[57] retrospectively studied outcomes in 46 patients with RV failure who received a TH-RVAD, of whom 21 patients were cannulated percutaneously. TH-RVAD implantation was associated with a significant decrease in RA pressure and a significant increase in CI. In-hospital mortality was 33% in patients with AMI. In another study by Kapur and colleagues,[58] 9 patients, 6 of whom had AMI, had improved hemodynamics when

Table 6
Major studies assessing acute mechanical circulatory support in right ventricular dysfunction

Study, Year Published	Device	Number of Patients	Population	Outcomes
Cheung et al,[55] 2014	Impella RP	18	39% AMI, other etiologies include post-transplant, myocarditis	30-d survival 72% 1-y survival 50% Hemodynamic effects: increased CI, decreased RA pressure
Anderson et al,[56] 2015	Impella RP	30	40% AMI, others include post-LVAD	30-d survival 73.3% Hemodynamic effects: increased CI, decreased RA pressure
Kapur et al,[57] 2013	TH-RVAD	46	25% AMI, others include post–cardiac surgery, transplant, myocarditis	In-hospital mortality 57% Hemodynamic effects: increased CI, MAP and PA, decreased RA pressure
Kapur et al,[58] 2011	TH-RVAD	9	66.7% AMI, others include post–cardiac surgery	In-hospital mortality 44% Hemodynamic effects: increased RV stroke volume, MAP and PA, decreased RA pressure
Truby et al,[65] 2015	VA-ECMO	179	26% AMI, others include post–cardiac surgery	In-hospital mortality 38.6% Hemodynamic effects: decreased RA and mean PA pressure

Abbreviations: MAP, mean arterial pressure; PA, pulmonary artery.

treated with TH-RVAD, with an in-hospital mortality rate of 44%.

SHOCK PROTOCOLS AND TEAMS

Shock protocols allow for a uniform treatment strategy in an effort to provide patients, nurses, and clinicians a systematic pathway of care,[59] although shock teams provide a diverse set of options that can be catered to the individual patient, taking into account operator and institutional expertise.[60] This concept is best exemplified in the work of the NCSI. Investigators involved in the study began by reviewing outcomes data in AMICS and forming best practices, which were put together into a shock protocol. The study was limited to evaluating outcomes in patients with AMICS and not other shock phenotypes. The study also used inclusion and exclusion criteria similar to previous RCTs in an effort to compare with prior work.

The shock protocol was piloted in metro Detroit and named the Detroit Cardiogenic Shock Initiative.[61] A 41-patient pilot study found

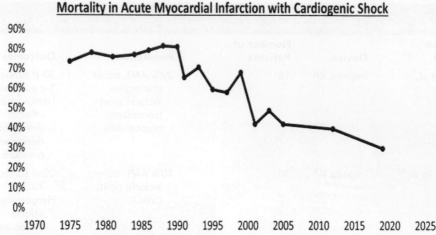

Mortality in Acute Myocardial Infarction with Cardiogenic Shock

Fig. 1. The 50-year mortality trend in AMI complicated by CS. Over 50 years, mortality in AMI with CS has increased steadily from approximately 80% to close to 30%. (*Adapted from* Goldberg RJ, Spencer FA, Gore JM, Lessard D, Yarzebski J. Thirty-year trends (1975 to 2005) in the magnitude of, management of, and hospital death rates associated with cardiogenic shock in patients with acute myocardial infarction: a population-based perspective. Circulation. 2009;119(9):1211-1219; with permission.)

the protocol could be used across selected centers and was associated with high survival compared with historical studies and local outcomes. The study then was expanded and renamed the NCSI. The goal was to see if the shock protocol could be reproduced in centers across the United States. In total, greater than 60 sites were recruited with a goal of enrolling 400 patients. The NCSI is the first contemporary study to evaluate outcomes of a shock protocol. The best practices included in the protocol are[1] to identify AMICS early and treat patients in the

catheterization laboratory (early is defined as <90 minutes to 120 minutes of diagnosis and prior to escalating use of inotropes)[2]; placement of Impella prior to PCI, because PCI can result in reperfusion injury, distal embolization, and transient cessation of coronary perfusion with balloon inflations and stents, which are better tolerated with MCS; and[3] use of pulmonary artery catheters to assess patients underlying hemodynamic state and to guide further therapy, including escalation of MCS, identification of RV failure, and weaning. The study has

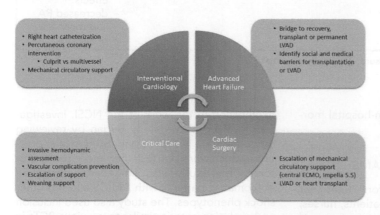

Fig. 2. Key components of a CS team. Using a shock team and protocol has been associated with improved outcomes in numerous observational studies. Early triage, prompt identification, and rapid delivery of MCS based on a patient's physiologic state are steps important in CS management. A multidisciplinary team–based approach, which includes interventional cardiology, advanced heart failure, cardiac surgery, and critical care, has proved efficient in improving outcomes without delaying care and it is highly recommended in clinical practice. Early identification of shock starts in the emergency department and the decision to send a patient to the catheterization laboratory should not be delayed, which highlights the importance of good communication between the emergency department and the cardiology team. Escalation for additional left ventricle or RV support as well as transfer to a tertiary care center (if needed) should be discussed early by the multidisciplinary team.

enrolled more than 300 patients with AMICS and has demonstrated survival to hospital discharge greater than 70%.[62,63]

SUMMARY

AMI complicated by CS is a deadly condition associated with significant morbidity and mortality (**Fig. 1**). Despite 20 years of medical advancements, early revascularization remains the sole therapy proved to improve outcomes. MCS devices provide a physiologically plausible mechanism of improving outcomes by offering hemodynamic stability for revascularization and improving end-organ perfusion. Results from well-powered RCTs, however, are not yet available. RCTs have been difficult to conduct in this patient population; until such trials are performed, implementing shock teams and protocols has been associated with improved outcomes in observational studies and may be considered (**Fig. 2**). Technological advancements will lead to continued development of more mobile, smaller-caliber, and more powerful MCS devices. Understanding the mechanism of action and physiologic effects of these devices, therefore, is critically important.

DISCLOSURE

M.B. Basir is a consultant for Abbott Vascular, Abiomed, Cardiovascular Systems, Chiesi, Procyrion and Zoll. A. Lemor and L. Ya'qoub report no conflicts of interest.

REFERENCES

1. Reynolds HR, Hochman JS. Cardiogenic shock: current concepts and improving outcomes. Circulation 2008;117(5):686–97.
2. Boyd JC, Cox JL, Hassan A, et al. Where you live in nova scotia can significantly impact your access to lifesaving cardiac care: access to invasive care influences survival. Can J Cardiol 2018;34(2):202–8.
3. Hochman JS, Sleeper LA, Webb JG, et al. Early revascularization in acute myocardial infarction complicated by cardiogenic shock. SHOCK Investigators. Should We Emergently Revascularize Occluded Coronaries for Cardiogenic Shock. N Engl J Med 1999;341(9):625–34.
4. Thiele H, Akin I, Sandri M, et al. PCI strategies in patients with acute myocardial infarction and cardiogenic shock. N Engl J Med 2017;377(25): 2419–32.
5. Garcia S, Schmidt CW, Garberich R, et al. Temporal changes in patient characteristics and outcomes in ST-segment elevation myocardial infarction 2003-

6. 2018. Catheter Cardiovasc Interv 2020. https://doi.org/10.1002/ccd.28901.
6. Rab T, O'Neill W. Mechanical circulatory support for patients with cardiogenic shock. Trends Cardiovasc Med 2019;29(7):410–7.
7. Parissis H, Graham V, Lampridis S, et al. IABP: history-evolution-pathophysiology-indications: what we need to know. J Cardiothorac Surg 2016; 11(1):122.
8. Dahlslett T, Karlsen S, Grenne B, et al. Intra-aortic balloon pump optimizes myocardial function during cardiogenic shock. JACC Cardiovasc Imaging 2018;11(3):512–4.
9. Moulopoulos S, Stamatelopoulos S, Petrou P. Intra-aortic balloon assistance in intractable cardiogenic shock. Eur Heart J 1986;7(5):396–403.
10. Bengtson JR, Kaplan AJ, Pieper KS, et al. Prognosis in cardiogenic shock after acute myocardial infarction in the interventional era. J Am Coll Cardiol 1992;20(7):1482–9.
11. Waksman R, Weiss AT, Gotsman MS, et al. Intra-aortic balloon counterpulsation improves survival in cardiogenic shock complicating acute myocardial infarction. Eur Heart J 1993;14(1):71–4.
12. Stomel RJ, Rasak M, Bates ER. Treatment strategies for acute myocardial infarction complicated by cardiogenic shock in a community hospital. Chest 1994;105(4):997–1002.
13. Anderson RD, Ohman EM, Holmes DR Jr, et al. Use of intraaortic balloon counterpulsation in patients presenting with cardiogenic shock: observations from the GUSTO-I Study—Global Utilization of Streptokinase and TPA for Occluded Coronary Arteries. J Am Coll Cardiol 1997;30(3):708–15.
14. Kovack PJ, Rasak MA, Bates ER, et al. Thrombolysis plus aortic counterpulsation: improved survival in patients who present to community hospitals with cardiogenic shock. J Am Coll Cardiol 1997;29(7): 1454–8.
15. Brodie BR, Stuckey TD, Hansen C, et al. Intra-aortic balloon counterpulsation before primary percutaneous transluminal coronary angioplasty reduces catheterization laboratory events in high-risk patients with acute myocardial infarction. Am J Cardiol 1999;84(1):18–23.
16. Kumbasar SD, Semiz E, Sancaktar O, et al. Concomitant use of intraaortic balloon counterpulsation and streptokinase in acute anterior myocardial infarction. Angiology 1999;50(6):465–71.
17. Sanborn TA, Sleeper LA, Bates ER, et al. Impact of thrombolysis, intra-aortic balloon pump counterpulsation, and their combination in cardiogenic shock complicating acute myocardial infarction: a report from the SHOCK Trial Registry—should we emergently revascularize occluded coronaries for cardiogenic shock? J Am Coll Cardiol 2000;36: 1123–9 (3)(suppl A).

18. Barron HV, Every NR, Parsons LS, et al. Investigators in the National Registry of Myocardial Infarction 2. The use of intra-aortic balloon counterpulsation in patients with cardiogenic shock complicating acute myocardial infarction: data from the National Registry of Myocardial Infarction 2. Am Heart J 2001;141(6):933–9.

19. Zeymer U, Bauer T, Hamm C, et al. Use and impact of intra-aortic balloon pump on mortality in patients with acute myocardial infarction complicated by cardiogenic shock: results of the Euro Heart Survey on PCI. EuroIntervention 2011;7(4):437–41.

20. Sjauw KD, Engström AE, Vis MM, et al. Efficacy and timing of intra-aortic counterpulsation in patients with ST-elevation myocardial infarction complicated by cardiogenic shock. Neth Heart J 2012; 20(10):402–9.

21. Zeymer U, Hochadel M, Hauptmann KE, et al. Intra-aortic balloon pump in patients with acute myocardial infarction complicated by cardiogenic shock: results of the ALKK-PCI registry. Clin Res Cardiol 2013;102(3):223–7.

22. Ohman EM, Nanas J, Stomel RJ, et al. Thrombolysis and counterpulsation to improve survival in myocardial infarction complicated by hypotension and suspected cardiogenic shock or heart failure: results of the TACTICS Trial. J Thromb Thrombolysis 2005;19(1):33–9.

23. Mandawat A, Rao SV. Percutaneous mechanical circulatory support devices in cardiogenic shock. Circ Cardiovasc Interv 2017;10(5):e004337.

24. Prondzinsky R, Lemm H, Swyter M, et al. Intra-aortic balloon counterpulsation in patients with acute myocardial infarction complicated by cardiogenic shock: the prospective, randomized IABP SHOCK Trial for attenuation of multiorgan dysfunction syndrome. Crit Care Med 2010;38:152–60.

25. Thiele H, Zeymer U, Neumann FJ, et al. Intraaortic balloon support for myocardial infarction with cardiogenic shock. N Engl J Med 2012;367(14): 1287–96.

26. Thiele H, Zeymer U, Thelemann N, et al. Intraaortic Balloon Pump in Cardiogenic Shock Complicating Acute Myocardial Infarction: Long-Term 6-Year Outcome of the Randomized IABP-SHOCK II Trial. Circulation 2018. https://doi.org/10.1161/CIRCULATIONAHA.118.038201.

27. Ahmad Y, Sen S, Shun-Shin MJ, et al. Intra-aortic balloon pump therapy for acute myocardial infarction: a meta-analysis. JAMA Intern Med 2015;175: 931–9.

28. Unverzagt S, Buerke M, de Waha A, et al. Intra-aortic balloon pump counterpulsation (IABP) for myocardial infarction complicated by cardiogenic shock. Cochrane Database Syst Rev 2015;(3):CD007398.

29. Rios SA, Bravo CA, Weinreich M, et al. Meta-Analysis and Trial Sequential Analysis Comparing Percutaneous Ventricular Assist Devices Versus Intra-Aortic Balloon Pump During High-Risk Percutaneous Coronary Intervention or Cardiogenic Shock. Am J Cardiol 2018;122(8):1330–8.

30. Ibanez B, James S, Agewall S, et al. 2017 ESC guidelines for the management of acute myocardial infarction in patients presenting with ST-segment elevation: the task force for the management of acute myocardial infarction in patients presenting with ST-segment elevation of the European Society of Cardiology (ESC). Eur Heart J 2018;39: 119–77.

31. O'Gara PT, Kushner FG, Ascheim DD, et al. American College of Cardiology Foundation/American Heart Association Task Force on Practice Guidelines. 2013 ACCF/AHA guideline for the management of ST-elevation myocardial infarction: a report of the American College of Cardiology Foundation/American Heart Association Task Force on Practice Guidelines. Circulation 2013; 127:e362–425.

32. Malick W, Fried JA, Masoumi A, et al. comparison of the hemodynamic response to intra-aortic balloon counterpulsation in patients with cardiogenic shock resulting from acute myocardial infarction versus acute decompensated heart failure. Am J Cardiol 2019;124(12):1947–53.

33. Vallabhajosyula S, Prasad A, Sandhu GS, et al. Mechanical circulatory support-assisted early percutaneous coronary intervention in acute myocardial infarction with cardiogenic shock: 10-year national temporal trends, predictors and outcomes. EuroIntervention 2019. https://doi.org/10.4244/EIJ-D-19-00226.

34. Keebler ME, Haddad EV, Choi CW, et al. Venoarterial extracorporeal membrane oxygenation in cardiogenic shock. JACC Heart Fail 2018;6(6): 503–16.

35. Sheu JJ, Tsai TH, Lee FY, et al. Early extracorporeal membrane oxygenator-assisted primary percutaneous coronary intervention improved 30-day clinical outcomes in patients with ST-segment elevation myocardial infarction complicated with profound cardiogenic shock. Crit Care Med 2010; 38(9):1810–7.

36. Esper SA, Bermudez C, Dueweke EJ, et al. Extracorporeal membrane oxygenation support in acute coronary syndromes complicated by cardiogenic shock. Catheter Cardiovasc Interv 2015;86(Suppl 1):S45–50.

37. Negi SI, Sokolovic M, Koifman E, et al. Contemporary use of veno-arterial extracorporeal membrane oxygenation for refractory cardiogenic shock in acute coronary syndrome. J Invasive Cardiol 2016; 28(2):52–7.

38. Vallabhajosyula S, Prasad A, Bell MR, et al. Extracorporeal membrane oxygenation use in acute myocardial infarction in the United States, 2000 to 2014. Circ Heart Fail 2019;12(12):e005929.

39. Gershlick A. EURO SHOCK testing the value of novel strategy and its cost efficacy in order to improve the poor outcomes in cardiogenic shock. ClinicalTrials.gov identifier: NCT03813134.

40. Thiele H. Prospective randomized multicenter study comparing extracorporeal life support plus optimal medical care versus optimal medical care alone in patients with acute myocardial infarction complicated by cardiogenic shock undergoing revascularization. ClinicalTrials.gov identifier: NCT03637205.

41. Kar B, Gregoric ID, Basra SS, et al. The percutaneous ventricular assist device in severe refractory cardiogenic shock. J Am Coll Cardiol 2011;57:688–96.

42. Smith L, Peters A, Mazimba S, et al. Outcomes of patients with cardiogenic shock treated with TandemHeart® percutaneous ventricular assist device: Importance of support indication and definitive therapies as determinants of prognosis. Catheter Cardiovasc Interv 2018;92(6):1173–81.

43. Thiele H, Sick P, Boudriot E, et al. Randomized comparison of intra-aortic balloon support with a percutaneous left ventricular assist device in patients with revascularized acute myocardial infarction complicated by cardiogenic shock. Eur Heart J 2005;26(13):1276–83.

44. Burkhoff D, Cohen H, Brunckhorst C, et al, TandemHeart Investigators Group. A randomized multicenter clinical study to evaluate the safety and efficacy of the TandemHeart percutaneous ventricular assist device versus conventional therapy with intraaortic balloon pumping for treatment of cardiogenic shock. Am Heart J 2006;152(3):469.e1-e8.

45. Lauten A, Engström AE, Jung C, et al. Percutaneous left-ventricular support with the Impella-2.5-assist device in acute cardiogenic shock: results of the Impella-EUROSHOCK-registry. Circ Heart Fail 2013;6(1):23–30.

46. Karatolios K, Chatzis G, Markus B, et al. Impella support compared to medical treatment for post-cardiac arrest shock after out of hospital cardiac arrest. Resuscitation 2018;126:104–10.

47. Schrage B, Ibrahim K, Loehn T, et al. Impella Support for Acute Myocardial Infarction Complicated by Cardiogenic Shock. Circulation 2019;139(10):1249–58.

48. Lemor A, Hosseini Dehkordi SH, Basir MB, et al. Impella versus extracorporeal membrane oxygenation for acute myocardial infarction cardiogenic shock [published online ahead of print, 2020 May 30]. Cardiovasc Revasc Med 2020. https://doi.org/10.1016/j.carrev.2020.05.042.

49. Loehn T, O'Neill WW, Lange B, et al. Long term survival after early unloading with Impella CP((R)) in acute myocardial infarction complicated by cardiogenic shock. Eur Heart J Acute Cardiovasc Care 2020;9(2):149–57.

50. Helgestad OKL, Josiassen J, Hassager C, et al. Contemporary trends in use of mechanical circulatory support in patients with acute MI and cardiogenic shock. Open Heart 2020;7(1):e001214.

51. Seyfarth M, Sibbing D, Bauer I, et al. A randomized clinical trial to evaluate the safety and efficacy of a percutaneous left ventricular assist device versus intra-aortic balloon pumping for treatment of cardiogenic shock caused by myocardial infarction. J Am Coll Cardiol 2008;52(19):1584–8.

52. Ouweneel DM, Eriksen E, Sjauw KD, et al. Percutaneous mechanical circulatory support versus intra-aortic balloon pump in cardiogenic shock after acute myocardial infarction. J Am Coll Cardiol 2017;69(3):278–87.

53. Lala A, Guo Y, Xu J, et al. Right ventricular dysfunction in acute myocardial infarction complicated by cardiogenic shock: a hemodynamic analysis of the should we emergently revascularize occluded coronaries for cardiogenic shock (SHOCK) Trial and Registry. J Card Fail 2018;24(3):148–56.

54. Jacobs AK, Leopold JA, Bates E, et al. Cardiogenic shock caused by right ventricular infarction: a report from the SHOCK registry. J Am Coll Cardiol 2003;41(8):1273–9.

55. Cheung AW, White CW, Davis MK, et al. Short-term mechanical circulatory support for recovery from acute right ventricular failure: clinical outcomes. J Heart Lung Transplant 2014;33:794–9.

56. Anderson MB, Goldstein J, Milano C, et al. Benefits of a novel percutaneous ventricular assist device for right heart failure: the prospective RECOVER RIGHT study of the Impella RP device. J Heart Lung Transplant 2015;34:1549–60.

57. Kapur NK, Paruchuri V, Jagannathan A, et al. Mechanical circulatory support for right ventricular failure. JACC Heart Fail 2013;1:127–34.

58. Kapur NK, Paruchuri V, Korabathina R, et al. Effects of a percutaneous mechanical circulatory support device for medically refractory right ventricular failure. J Heart Lung Transplant 2011;30:1360–7.

59. Basir MB, Kapur NK, Patel K, et al. Improved Outcomes Associated with the use of Shock Protocols: Updates from the National Cardiogenic Shock Initiative. Catheter Cardiovasc Interv 2019;93(7):1173–83.

60. Tehrani BN, Truesdell AG, Sherwood MW, et al. Standardized Team-Based Care for Cardiogenic Shock. J Am Coll Cardiol 2019;73(13):1659–69.

61. Basir MB, Schreiber T, Dixon S, et al. Feasibility of early mechanical circulatory support in acute myocardial infarction complicated by cardiogenic shock: The Detroit cardiogenic shock initiative. Catheter Cardiovasc Interv 2018;91(3):454–61. https://doi.org/10.1002/ccd.27427.

62. Hanson ID, Tagami T, Mando R, et al. National Cardiogenic Shock Investigators. SCAI shock classification in acute myocardial infarction: Insights from the National Cardiogenic Shock Initiative. Catheter Cardiovasc Interv 2020. https://doi.org/10.1002/ccd.29139.

63. Lemor A, Basir MB, Patel K, et al. National cardiogenic shock initiative investigators. multivessel versus culprit-vessel percutaneous coronary intervention in cardiogenic shock. JACC Cardiovasc Interv 2020;13(10):1171–8.

64. Taleb I, Koliopoulou AG, Tandar A, et al. Shock team approach in refractory cardiogenic shock requiring short-term mechanical circulatory support: a proof of concept. Circulation 2019;140(1):98–100. https://doi.org/10.1161/CIRCULATIONAHA.119.040654.

65. Truby L, Mundy L, Kalesan B, et al. Contemporary outcomes of venoarterial extracorporeal membrane oxygenation for refractory cardiogenic shock at a large tertiary care center. ASAIO J 2015;61(4):403–9. https://doi.org/10.1097/MAT.0000000000000225.

Mechanical Circulatory Support in Right Ventricular Failure

Akbarshakh Akhmerov, MD[a], Danny Ramzy, MD, PhD[b],*

KEYWORDS

• Right ventricular failure • Right ventricular assist device • Impella • Tandem

KEY POINTS

- The right ventricle is distinct from the left ventricle in anatomy, physiology, and pathophysiology.
- The failed right ventricle is challenging to manage and is associated with higher mortality.
- Short-term percutaneous devices can be used to support the right ventricle but require careful selection.

INTRODUCTION

Right heart failure is a clinical syndrome that arises from dysfunction in any of the components constituting the right-sided circulatory system.[1] This system includes all the elements between the systemic venous and pulmonary circulations: systemic veins, right atrium, coronary sinus, tricuspid valve, right ventricle (RV), pulmonic valve, and pulmonary circulation up to the capillary bed. For the purposes of this review, we will focus only on cardiopulmonary causes of right heart failure, with specific attention given to RV dysfunction.

The prevalence of RV dysfunction is difficult to ascertain, given the variability in reported populations, but typically ranges from 47% to 76% in heart failure with reduced ejection fraction (HFrEF) and from 33% to 50% in heart failure with preserved ejection fraction (HFpEF).[2–5] In both settings, the presence of RV dysfunction confers an increased risk of morbidity and mortality. The association between RV dysfunction and increased mortality has been demonstrated in acute myocardial infarction (AMI),[6–10] myocarditis,[11,12] postcardiotomy cardiogenic shock

(PCCS),[13] left ventricular assist device (LVAD) implantation,[14] cardiac transplantation,[13] transplant rejection,[15] pulmonary embolism,[16,17] pulmonary arterial hypertension,[18,19] and many others.[20] Thus, RV dysfunction appears to be both prevalent and prognostic in cardiopulmonary disease.

In this review, we discuss the RV in the context of normal function and dysfunction and present therapeutic strategies with the primary focus on mechanical circulatory support (MCS).

THE RIGHT VENTRICLE IN HEALTH AND DISEASE

Anatomy

The RV differs from the left ventricle (LV) embryologically, anatomically, and physiologically. The RV is derived from the secondary heart field (in contrast to LV, which is derived from the primary heart field), and develops into a thin-walled, crescent-shaped chamber.[20] And although the RV chamber is 10% to 15% larger in volume compared with the LV, it is only one-sixth its mass.[21–23] Anatomically, the RV can be divided into 3 regions: (1) the inlet region, containing the tricuspid valve, chordae tendinae, and ≥ 3

Funding: A. Akhmerov was funded by the National Institutes of Health (NIH) T32HL116273-07 (Training in Advanced Heart Disease Research).
[a] Department of Cardiac Surgery, Smidt Heart Institute, Cedars-Sinai Medical Center, 127 S. San Vicente Boulevard, Suite A3105, Los Angeles, CA 90048, USA; [b] Department of Cardiac Surgery, Smidt Heart Institute, Cedars-Sinai Medical Center, 127 S. San Vicente Boulevard, Suite A3105, Los Angeles, CA 90048, USA
* Corresponding author.
E-mail address: danny.ramzy@cshs.org

papillary muscles, (2) the trabeculated apex, and (3) the muscular infundibulum, corresponding with the outflow tract.[21] The RV can be further distinguished from the LV based on the architecture of its myofibers. Unlike the LV, which is composed of 3 muscular layers, the RV is composed of 2 layers: a superficial layer and a deep layer. The superficial myofibers are arranged circumferentially and roughly parallel to the atrioventricular groove, whereas the deeper myofibers are arranged longitudinally along the axis between the base and apex.[21] Shortening of the longitudinal fibers accounts for the majority of RV contraction.[24] Despite the different myofiber arrangements between the LV and RV, there is continuity of fibers between the two ventricles, which, along with the interventricular septum, accounts for the ventricular interdependence.

Physiology

Unlike the LV, the RV is highly compliant and ejects stroke volume into a low resistance pulmonary system. Owing to the low impedance of the pulmonary system, the RV's overall stroke work is only 25% of the LV, even with the same stroke volumes.[22,25] Thus, the RV is a well-suited conduit between the systemic venous and pulmonary circulations. The unique features of the RV under normal physiologic conditions, as well as pathophysiology, can be best understood in terms of contractility, preload, and afterload. The contractility and afterload can be approximated from the RV pressure-volume loops using a time varying elastance model.[26] In this model, the end-systolic elastance (E_{es}) and arterial elastance (E_a) correspond with contractility and afterload, respectively. On a pressure–volume loop for the RV, the E_{es} is derived from the slope of varying end-systolic pressure–volume relations, and the E_a is derived from the slope connecting the end-systolic and end-diastolic volumes (Fig. 1A). In analysis of RV systolic function and dysfunction, the E_{es}/E_a ratio, known as ventriculoarterial coupling, is instructive.[27] This ratio allows an assessment of RV function relative to its load, and a ratio of $E_{es}/E_a \approx 1.5$ to 2.0 represents an optimal and efficient flow from the RV. In the setting of pathology, adaptive responses attempt to maintain or restore ventriculoarterial coupling. For example, during increased afterload, one of the initial responses is the thickening of the myocardial wall, which, according to LaPlace's law, decreases wall stress and restores coupling. In progressive disease, however, the RV ultimately dilates and fails, resulting in ventriculoarterial uncoupling ($E_{es}/E_a \leq 1.3$).[27,28]

The RV function also depends on preload, following the basic Frank–Starling mechanism. Under normal physiologic conditions, the RV is highly compliant and can accommodate varying degrees of preload. In instances of excessive preload, however, the RV can impinge upon the LV and thereby diminish cardiac output (CO) (ventricular interdependence). Given its high compliance, this excess in RV preload would need to be substantial. On the other hand, the RV is highly susceptible to changes in afterload, with relatively small changes in pulmonary artery (PA) pressure, leading to large shifts in RV stroke volume (Fig. 1B).[29] Therefore, afterload is the primary determinant of normal RV function.[20] These hemodynamic considerations (ie, contractility, preload, and afterload) are also vital to understanding the pathophysiology of RV dysfunction.

Right Ventricular Dysfunction and Treatment

Right heart failure can result from a wide variety of causes, both intrinsic and extrinsic to the heart. The most common intrinsic cause is left heart failure. Other causes include MI and valvular disease. Extrinsic causes include pulmonary parenchymal and pulmonary vascular diseases. Acute respiratory distress syndrome, chronic obstructive pulmonary disease, and interstitial lung disease are examples of parenchymal causes, whereas acute pulmonary embolism and pulmonary hypertension represent vascular causes. For heuristic purposes, these etiologies can also be grouped according to whether they affect preload, afterload, or contractility. For example, left heart failure, pulmonic stenosis, and pulmonary disease affect afterload; valvular regurgitation, congenital heart disease, and LVADs influence preload; and MI, primary cardiomyopathies, and postcardiotomy shock affect contractility (Fig. 2).

Manifestations of right heart failure may include notable physical examination findings (eg, hypotension, tachycardia, jugular vein distension, and peripheral edema); serum marker elevations (eg, cardiac troponin, brain natriuretic peptide, creatinine, and transaminases); or electrocardiographic abnormalities (eg, right axis deviation, right bundle branch block, ST segment elevations in V4R, and the S1Q3T3 pattern).[30,31] These indicators, however, are often nonspecific and do not confirm RV dysfunction. A definitive diagnosis requires echocardiographic and invasive hemodynamic assessment. On echocardiography, RV function is evaluated using tricuspid annular plane systolic excursion (<1.6 cm), RV fractional area change (<35%), RV outflow tract acceleration (<100 ms), and tricuspid

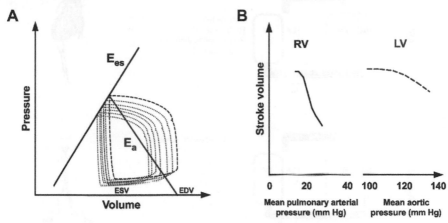

Fig. 1. Physiology of the right ventricle. (A) The pressure-volume loop of the right ventricle depicts the end-systolic elastance (Ees) in *blue*, derived from the slope of varying end-systolic pressure-volume relations, and the arterial elastance (Ea) in *red*, derived from the slope connecting the end-systolic and end-diastolic volumes. (B) Changes in RV stroke volume *in blue* and LV stroke volume *in red* in relation to changes in afterload. The afterload is determined by the mean pulmonary artery pressure for the RV and the mean aortic pressure for the LV (x axis). (*Adapted from* Konstam MA, Kiernan MS, Bernstein D, et al. Evaluation and management of right-sided heart failure: a scientific statement from the American Heart Association. Circulation 2018;137(20):e578–622. [Created with Bio-Render.com.])

regurgitation jet velocity, in addition to other parameters.[20] Hemodynamic assessment with a PA catheter can be both diagnostic and prognostic. For example, elevated right atrial (RA) to pulmonary capillary wedge pressure (PCWP) ratios can predict RV failure, with an RA/PCWP ratio of greater than 0.63 predicting failure after LVAD placement and an RA/PCWP of greater than 0.86 predicting failure after AMI.[32,33] The ratio of the PA pulse pressure to RA pressure (or the PA pulsatility index) is also a useful and predictive marker for right heart failure (PA pulsatility index of <1.85 for LVAD placement; PA pulsatility index of <1.0 in MI).[34,35]

Once the diagnosis of RV dysfunction is established, therapy includes treatment of the underlying pathology and optimizing cardiac function. The treatment of underlying causes may include coronary revascularization, pulmonary embolism management (thrombolytics, mechanical or surgical thrombectomy),[36] and other definitive interventions. Optimizing cardiac function includes (1) addressing preload with either fluids or diuretics, depending on the volume status (goal central venous pressure of 12–15 mm Hg), (2) addressing afterload with either inhaled pulmonary vasodilators, adjustments in mechanical ventilation, or management of LV failure, and (3) addressing

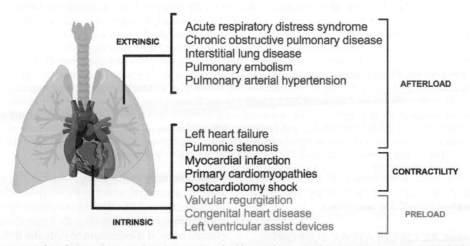

Fig. 2. Causes of RV failure. Causes of RV failure classified by etiology as either intrinsic or extrinsic to the heart and according to whether they affect afterload (*red*), contractility (*blue*), or preload (*green*). Etiologies of RV failure can affect multiple physiologic processes simultaneously. (Created with BioRender.com.)

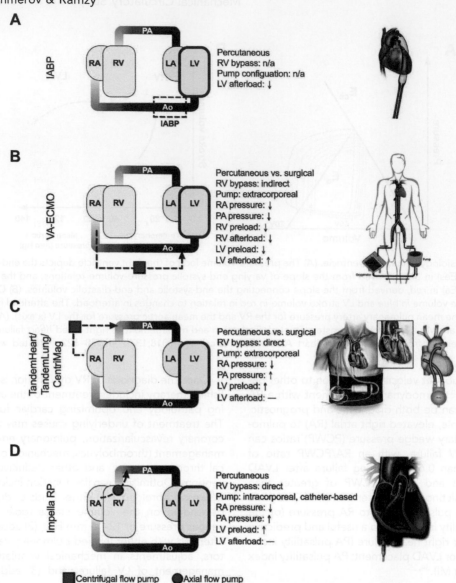

Fig. 3. MCS devices for RV failure. Mechanical assist devices for RV failure include (*A*) intra-aortic balloon pumps, (*B*) veno-arterial extracorporeal membrane oxygenation, (*C*) TandemHeart, TandemLung, and CentriMag devices; and (*D*) Impella RP. These devices are deployed percutaneously or surgically, have axial flow or centrifugal flow pumps, bypass RV directly or indirectly, and are associated with distinct hemodynamic profiles. IABP, intra-aortic balloon pump; VA-ECMO, veno-arterial extracorporeal membrane oxygenation. (*Adapted from* Dell'Italia LJ, Starling MR, O'Rourke RA. Physical examination for exclusion of hemodynamically important right ventricular infarction. Ann Intern Med 1983;99(5):608–11, Kapur NK, Esposito ML, Bader Y, et al. Mechanical circulatory support devices for acute right ventricular failure. Circulation 2017;136(3):314–26, Sultan I, Kilic A, Kilic A. Short-term circulatory and right ventricle support in cardiogenic shock: extracorporeal membrane oxygenation, tandem CentriMag, and Impella. Heart Fail Clin 2018;14(4):579–83, and Anderson MB, Goldstein J, Milano C, et al. Benefits of a novel percutaneous ventricular assist device for right heart failure: the prospective RECOVER RIGHT study of the Impella RP device. J Heart Lung Transplant 2015;34(12):1549–60. [Created with BioRender.com.])

contractility with vasopressor and/or inotropic support. If optimal medical therapy fails, then consideration for MCS is warranted.

MECHANICAL CIRCULATORY SUPPORT

The MCS devices discussed in this article can be classified according to whether they are deployed

percutaneously or surgically, whether the pump is axial or centrifugal, whether RV is bypassed directly or indirectly, and whether the duration of support is short term or long term (**Fig. 3**). Regardless of the classification, it is important to note the differences and similarities among different devices, along with the relative advantages and disadvantages associated with each device. The choice of the most appropriate device depends on patient-specific needs and center-specific capabilities.

Intra-Aortic Balloon Pump

Intra-aortic balloon pumps (IABPs) are among the most widely used mechanical support devices, but their role in isolated RV dysfunction is uncertain. The device is implanted percutaneously, most commonly via the common femoral artery, and positioned within the proximal descending thoracic aorta (see Fig. 3A). The balloon inflates after the closure of the aortic valve and deflates immediately before its opening, thereby augmenting coronary perfusion in diastole and decreasing afterload during systole.[37,38] In RV failure, IABP support may be beneficial in the setting of postcardiotomy cardiogenic shock (PCCS), post-transplant allograft dysfunction, and AMI. In retrospective studies of PCCS and allograft dysfunction with predominant RV failure, the initiation of IABP resulted in increased cardiac index and mean arterial pressure; and decreased central venous pressure and PA wedge pressure.[39,40] In a preclinical model of AMI, the use of IABP seemed to restore ventriculoarterial coupling, resulting in improved CO and mean arterial pressure. The RV contractility, however, did not appear to improve.[41] In preclinical models of acute RV failure owing to pressure overload, IABP support alone showed limited impact on hemodynamics, but may be beneficial when combined with vasopressors.[42,43] Unfortunately, no robust clinical data are available that demonstrate similar effects in patients. Therefore, although IABPs are relatively easy to implant and manage, their therapeutic role in RV dysfunction is limited.

Extracorporeal Membrane Oxygenation

Extracorporeal membrane oxygenation (ECMO) can be deployed for various etiologies of right heart failure, including isolated RV dysfunction, LV dysfunction, and pulmonary disease. For obstructive diseases involving the pulmonary circulation, ECMO may be the more appropriate strategy compared with right ventricular assist devices (RVADs), which can exacerbate elevations in the PA pressure (PAP).[20,44] Regardless of the etiology, the typical ECMO configuration is venoarterial ECMO (VA-ECMO). This configuration is achieved via percutaneous or surgical cannulation of the femoral vein and artery and provides an indirect RV bypass (see Fig. 3B). In this configuration, blood is drained from the right atrium and recirculated using an extracorporeal centrifugal pump and a membrane oxygenator.

It should be noted that an alternative veno-veno-arterial configuration can place inflow cannulas within the RA and PA. Physiologically, VA-ECMO decreases RA and PA pressures, decreases RV preload and afterload, and decreases LV preload (see Fig. 3B). The total peripheral resistance and LV afterload, however, are increased. Thus, in the setting of concomitant LV failure, CO will decrease and LV filling pressures will increase, with subsequent pulmonary edema and elevated PAPs.[45] To mitigate this event, an IABP, a decompressive left atrial/ventricular vent, or a temporary LV assist device can be placed.[46,47] Atrial septostomy is also an option.

Although clinical outcomes data are limited, VA-ECMO has been described in several important contexts of RV failure. In patients with RV dysfunction after LVAD placement, VA-ECMO support is associated with improved RV function, decreased central venous pressure and PAP, and increased CO. Ninety-one percent of patients are successfully weaned from ECMO and the 1-year survival is 75%.[48] Smaller case series show similar beneficial effects of VA-ECMO in patients with RV dysfunction secondary to LV failure and MI.[49–51] ECMO is clearly a suitable strategy for short-term support (<14 days)[52] and as a bridge therapy, especially in the setting of cardiopulmonary collapse or biventricular failure.

TandemHeart

The TandemHeart is a short-term, percutaneous RVAD driven by an extracorporeal centrifugal pump providing up to 4 L/min of flow. Unlike VA-ECMO, the TandemHeart provides direct RV bypass by diverting blood from the RA to the main PA.[45] To achieve this, the inflow cannula is typically placed into the RA via left femoral vein cannulation, and the outflow cannula is placed into the main PA via right femoral vein cannulation (see Fig. 3C). Alternatively, a single right internal jugular vein access can be used to deploy the Protek Duo dual-lumen coaxial cannula, which allows greater mobility and patient ambulation (see Fig. 3C).[53] The diversion of blood directly from the RA into PA confers a distinct hemodynamic profile, characterized by a decreased RA pressure, increased PAP, and increased LV preload (see Fig. 3C). In contrast with VA-ECMO, the LV afterload is not affected. With increased LV preload, the CO output is expected to increase, but in the setting of LV failure, the increased preload can result in elevated LV filling pressures and pulmonary edema. Thus, a circumspect approach is required to determine the optimal MCS strategy in biventricular failure.[54] If needed, LV unloading can be achieved using the techniques described for VA-ECMO.

Clinical data demonstrate both the feasibility and effectiveness of the TandemHeart in RV failure.[55,56] In a retrospective review of 46 patients with RV dysfunction, TandemHeart support was associated with improved hemodynamic status. The distribution for these patients were AMI (n = 12), myocarditis (n = 3), chronic left heart failure (n = 3), PCCS (n = 18), postcardiac transplantation (n = 5), and post-LVAD implantation (n = 5). However, the overall in-hospital mortality was 57%. Similarly, in a smaller cohort of patients with the Protek Duo (n = 17), the mortality rate was 41%.[57] Other studies with the TandemHeart and Protek Duo cannula demonstrate encouraging results. In a cohort of 20 patients with RV failure (post-LVAD implantation, n = 16; PCCS, n = 2; postcardiac transplantation, n = 2), the TandemHeart with Protek Duo support resulted in rapid decrease of inotropic support, with a 30-day survival rate of 80%.[58] Results clearly show that the TandemHeart RVAD has emerged as a promising MCS strategy.

TandemLung

The circuit described for the TandemHeart can be further modified to include an oxygenator, thereby providing simultaneous respiratory and hemodynamic support.[59] This iteration involves the TandemHeart extracorporeal centrifugal pump, the TandemLung oxygenator, and the Protek Duo cannula. Placement is via right internal jugular vein access. The oxygenator consists of a hollow fiber membrane with blood inflow and outflow ports, along with gas inlet and outlet ports. Priming requires only 240 mL of volume and is further simplified by the availability of a priming tray. Therefore, priming can be achieved without a perfusionist, offering an ideal option for non–perfusion-run ECMO centers. The maximal flow depends on the size of Protek Duo cannulae, which are available in 29F and 31F configurations. The 29F draining cannula returns the oxygenated blood via a 16F cannula into the PA, with a maximal flow of 4.5 L/min. The 31F draining cannula returns the blood via a 19F cannula with a maximal flow of 5 L/min. As mentioned elsewhere in this article for the TandemHeart, the deployment of the Tandem-Lung can be achieved percutaneously, and the use of the Protek Duo cannula allows ambulatory support. This contrasts with the CentriMag system (described elsewhere in this article), which requires open surgical deployment, and the Impella RP (described elsewhere in this article),

which requires femoral cannulation and precludes ambulatory support. Furthermore, the Impella RP is only capable of providing flows of up to 4 L/min. Finally, the Protek Duo cannula contrasts favorably against the bicaval, dual-lumen Avalon Elite cannula used in ECMO. Unlike the Avalon Elite system, the Protek Duo (1) allows for RV support during VV-ECMO, (2) eliminates recirculation and mixing, and (3) facilitates mobility and ambulation, given the greater positional stability of the cannula.

CentriMag

The CentriMag is an extracorporeal RVAD that utilizes a magnetically levitated centrifugal pump. In contrast with the percutaneous deployment of the TandemHeart, the CentriMag system requires surgical placement, either through a full sternotomy, thoracotomy, or minithoracotomy.[52,60,61] The diversion of blood and subsequent hemodynamic changes are similar to those of the Tandem-Heart (see Fig. 3C), but the major advantage of the CentriMag system is the ability to deliver flows of up to 10 L/min. However, the open surgical technique is associated with an additional risk of infection and bleeding.[62] These compounding dilemmas yield no simple answers in the selection of the optimal MCS. Clearly, clinical judgment with consideration of risks and benefits must guide the appropriate selection of MCS in all cases. Clinical studies of the CentriMag system will also inform this decision. Although robust outcomes data are not yet available, retrospective studies demonstrate the feasibility of using CentriMag in RV failure. These studies show weaning rates up to 59% and early mortality rates of 48% to 53%.[62,63] Further research is needed to identify optimal candidates for this MCS system.

Impella RP

The Impella RP device is a catheter-based, microaxial pump capable of providing short-term support with flow rates of up to 4 L/min. Deployed percutaneously, typically through femoral vein access, the inflow segment is positioned in the inferior vena cava and the outflow segment in the main PA. Thus, the pump extends through both the tricuspid and pulmonic valves and, like the TandemHeart RVAD, directly bypasses the RV (see Fig. 3D). Hemodynamic changes are also similar to the TandemHeart. After initiation of Impella RP, the RA pressures decrease, and the PAP and LV preloads increase (see Fig. 3D). There are no changes in LV afterload, and so in a normally functioning LV, the CO also increases. However, in the failing LV, the increased LV preload can result in greater filling pressures and pulmonary edema. Similar decompressive strategies can be used to relieve the LV as described for VA-ECMO. Compared with the TandemHeart or VA-ECMO, the deployment and management of the Impella RP is relatively easy,[64,65] and the risk of limb ischemia and anticoagulation requirements are lower. In contrast with VA-ECMO and the TandemHeart, however, there is no capability to splice in an oxygenator. This means that the device provides only hemodynamic support. Yet, despite this limitation, clinical outcomes with the Impella RP are promising.

In the initial prospective single-arm clinical trial (RECOVER RIGHT), 30 patients were supported with the Impella RP (18 with RV dysfunction after LVAD implantation and 12 with RV dysfunction after cardiotomy or MI). Initiation of the Impella RP was associated with significant improvements in the cardiac index and central venous pressure. An overall survival rate of 73% at 30 days was achieved.[66] More recently, a prospective cohort of 60 patients was investigated (31 with RV dysfunction after LVAD implantation and 29 with RV dysfunction after cardiotomy, heart transplant, or MI). Similar results were achieved, with significant improvements in the cardiac index and central venous pressure, and a 72% survival at 30 days or at the time of discharge.[67] These data demonstrate both hemodynamic efficacy and encouraging short-term survival.

SUMMARY

Our discussion has focused on devices optimally suited for short-term support. In patients who do not recover RV function, long-term devices, such as the total artificial heart, or conventional durable LVADs (eg, HeartWare, HeartMate 3, used in an off-label manner), are required.[68–71] It must be noted, however, that the optimal therapy for these patients is cardiac transplantation.

The RV is distinct from the LV in its anatomy, physiology, and pathophysiology. Because of its distinct complexities, the failed RV is challenging to manage and is associated with a higher risk of mortality. Acute MCS provides an effective, temporizing therapy in confronting advanced disease. As MCS technology continues to improve, temporary devices will become safer and more portable. Additional effective, long-term devices for the RV will emerge. Future research in this area will optimize device management, refine patient selection, and ultimately improve clinical outcomes.

CLINICS CARE POINTS

- The diagnosis of RV failure relies on echocardiographic and invasive hemodynamic assessment.
- The management of RV failure begins with treatment of underlying causes and medical optimization of cardiac function (preload, afterload, and contractility).
- In medically refractory patients, MCS should be considered.
- ECMO, TandemHeart, TandemLung, Impella RP, and CentriMag have unique hemodynamic profiles, and each device configuration has advantages and disadvantages.
- Selection of an MCS device will depend on patient-specific needs and center-specific capabilities.

DISCLOSURE

D. Ramzy is a speaker for Abiomed and LivaNova.

REFERENCES

1. Mehra MR, Park MH, Landzberg MJ, et al, International Right Heart Failure Foundation Scientific Working Group. Right heart failure: toward a common language. J Heart Lung Transplant 2014;33(2): 123–6.

2. Iglesias-Garriz I, Olalla-Gomez C, Garrote C, et al. Contribution of right ventricular dysfunction to heart failure mortality: a meta-analysis. Rev Cardiovasc Med 2012;13(2–3):e62–9.

3. Melenovsky V, Hwang SJ, Lin G, et al. Right heart dysfunction in heart failure with preserved ejection fraction. Eur Heart J 2014;35(48):3452–62.

4. Puwanant S, Priester TC, Mookadam F, et al. Right ventricular function in patients with preserved and reduced ejection fraction heart failure. Eur J Echocardiogr 2009;10(6):733–7.

5. Mohammed SF, Hussain I, AbouEzzeddine OF, et al. Right ventricular function in heart failure with preserved ejection fraction: a community-based study. Circulation 2014;130(25):2310–20.

6. Shah PK, Maddahi J, Staniloff HM, et al. Variable spectrum and prognostic implications of left and right ventricular ejection fractions in patients with and without clinical heart failure after acute myocardial infarction. Am J Cardiol 1986;58(6): 387–93.

7. Lim ST, Goldstein JA. Right ventricular infarction. Curr Treat Options Cardiovasc Med 2001;3(2): 95–101.

8. Mehta SR, Eikelboom JW, Natarajan MK, et al. Impact of right ventricular involvement on mortality

and morbidity in patients with inferior myocardial infarction. J Am Coll Cardiol 2001;37(1):37–43.

9. Zehender M, Kasper W, Kauder E, et al. Right ventricular infarction as an independent predictor of prognosis after acute inferior myocardial infarction. N Engl J Med 1993;328(14):981–8.

10. Serrano Junior CV, Ramires JA, Cesar LA, et al. Prognostic significance of right ventricular dysfunction in patients with acute inferior myocardial infarction and right ventricular involvement. Clin Cardiol 1995;18(4):199–205.

11. Mendes LA, Dec GW, Picard MH, et al. Right ventricular dysfunction: an independent predictor of adverse outcome in patients with myocarditis. Am Heart J 1994;128(2):301–7.

12. Caforio AL, Calabrese F, Angelini A, et al. A prospective study of biopsy-proven myocarditis: prognostic relevance of clinical and aetiopathogenetic features at diagnosis. Eur Heart J 2007; 28(11):1326–33.

13. Haddad F, Couture P, Tousignant C, et al. The right ventricle in cardiac surgery, a perioperative perspective: II. Pathophysiology, clinical importance, and management. Anesth Analg 2009; 108(2):422–33.

14. Kirklin JK, Naftel DC, Pagani FD, et al. Seventh INTERMACS annual report: 15,000 patients and counting. J Heart Lung Transplant 2015;34(12): 1495–504.

15. Haddad F, Fisher P, Pham M, et al. Right ventricular dysfunction predicts poor outcome following hemodynamically compromising rejection. J Heart Lung Transplant 2009;28(4):312–9.

16. Sanchez O, Planquette B, Roux A, et al. Triaging in pulmonary embolism. Semin Respir Crit Care Med 2012;33(2):156–62.

17. Coutance G, Cauderlier E, Ehtisham J, et al. The prognostic value of markers of right ventricular dysfunction in pulmonary embolism: a meta-analysis. Crit Care 2011;15(2):R103.

18. Chin KM, Kim NH, Rubin LJ. The right ventricle in pulmonary hypertension. Coron Artery Dis 2005; 16(1):13–8.

19. van de Veerdonk MC, Kind T, Marcus JT, et al. Progressive right ventricular dysfunction in patients with pulmonary arterial hypertension responding to therapy. J Am Coll Cardiol 2011; 58(24):2511–9.

20. Konstam MA, Kiernan MS, Bernstein D, et al. Evaluation and management of right-sided heart failure: a scientific statement from the American Heart Association. Circulation 2018;137(20):e578–622.

21. Haddad F, Hunt SA, Rosenthal DN, et al. Right ventricular function in cardiovascular disease, part I: anatomy, physiology, aging, and functional

assessment of the right ventricle. Circulation 2008; 117(11):1436–48.

22. Sanz J, Sanchez-Quintana D, Bossone E, et al. Anatomy, function, and dysfunction of the right ventricle: JACC state-of-the-art review. J Am Coll Cardiol 2019;73(12):1463–82.

23. Lorenz CH, Walker ES, Morgan VL, et al. Normal human right and left ventricular mass, systolic function, and gender differences by cine magnetic resonance imaging. J Cardiovasc Magn Reson 1999;1(1):7–21.

24. Brown SB, Raina A, Katz D, et al. Longitudinal shortening accounts for the majority of right ventricular contraction and improves after pulmonary vasodilator therapy in normal subjects and patients with pulmonary arterial hypertension. Chest 2011; 140(1):27–33.

25. Dell'Italia LJ. The right ventricle: anatomy, physiology, and clinical importance. Curr Probl Cardiol 1991;16(10):653–720.

26. Dell'Italia LJ, Walsh RA. Application of a time varying elastance model to right ventricular performance in man. Cardiovasc Res 1988;22(12):864–74.

27. Zelt JGE, Chaudhary KR, Cadete VJ, et al. Medical therapy for heart failure associated with pulmonary hypertension. Circ Res 2019;124(11):1551–67.

28. Vonk Noordegraaf A, Westerhof BE, Westerhof N. The relationship between the right ventricle and its load in pulmonary hypertension. J Am Coll Cardiol 2017;69(2):236–43.

29. MacNee W. Pathophysiology of cor pulmonale in chronic obstructive pulmonary disease. Part One. Am J Respir Crit Care Med 1994;150(3):833–52.

30. Dell'Italia LJ, Starling MR, O'Rourke RA. Physical examination for exclusion of hemodynamically important right ventricular infarction. Ann Intern Med 1983;99(5):608–11.

31. Matthews JC, McLaughlin V. Acute right ventricular failure in the setting of acute pulmonary embolism or chronic pulmonary hypertension: a detailed review of the pathophysiology, diagnosis, and management. Curr Cardiol Rev 2008;4(1):49–59.

32. Kormos RL, Teuteberg JJ, Pagani FD, et al. Right ventricular failure in patients with the HeartMate II continuous-flow left ventricular assist device: incidence, risk factors, and effect on outcomes. J Thorac Cardiovasc Surg 2010;139(5):1316–24.

33. Lopez-Sendon J, Coma-Canella I, Gamallo C. Sensitivity and specificity of hemodynamic criteria in the diagnosis of acute right ventricular infarction. Circulation 1981;64(3):515–25.

34. Morine KJ, Kiernan MS, Pham DT, et al. Pulmonary artery pulsatility index is associated with right ventricular failure after left ventricular assist device surgery. J Card Fail 2016;22(2):110–6.

35. Korabathina R, Heffernan KS, Paruchuri V, et al. The pulmonary artery pulsatility index identifies severe

right ventricular dysfunction in acute inferior myocardial infarction. Catheter Cardiovasc Interv 2012;80(4):593–600.

36. Akhmerov A, Reich H, Mirocha J, et al. Effect of percutaneous suction thromboembolectomy on improved right ventricular function. Tex Heart Inst J 2019;46(2):115–9.

37. Mueller H, Ayres SM, Conklin EF, et al. The effects of intra-aortic counterpulsation on cardiac performance and metabolism in shock associated with acute myocardial infarction. J Clin Invest 1971; 50(9):1885–900.

38. Kern MJ, Aguirre FV, Tatineni S, et al. Enhanced coronary blood flow velocity during intraaortic balloon counterpulsation in critically ill patients. J Am Coll Cardiol 1993;21(2):359–68.

39. Arafa OE, Geiran OR, Andersen K, et al. Intraaortic balloon pumping for predominantly right ventricular failure after heart transplantation. Ann Thorac Surg 2000;70(5):1587–93.

40. Boeken U, Feindt P, Litmathe J, et al. Intraaortic balloon pumping in patients with right ventricular insufficiency after cardiac surgery: parameters to predict failure of IABP Support. Thorac Cardiovasc Surg 2009;57(6):324–8.

41. Nordhaug D, Steensrud T, Muller S, et al. Intra-aortic balloon pumping improves hemodynamics and right ventricular efficiency in acute ischemic right ventricular failure. Ann Thorac Surg 2004; 78(4):1426–32.

42. Vanden Eynden F, Mets G, De Somer F, et al. Is there a place for intra-aortic balloon counterpulsation support in acute right ventricular failure by pressure-overload? Int J Cardiol 2015;197:227–34.

43. Liakopoulos OJ, Ho JK, Yezbick AB, et al. Right ventricular failure resulting from pressure overload: role of intra-aortic balloon counterpulsation and vasopressor therapy. J Surg Res 2010;164(1):58–66.

44. Verbelen T, Verhoeven J, Goda M, et al. Mechanical support of the pressure overloaded right ventricle: an acute feasibility study comparing low and high flow support. Am J Physiol Heart Circ Physiol 2015;309(4):H615–24.

45. Kapur NK, Esposito ML, Bader Y, et al. Mechanical circulatory support devices for acute right ventricular failure. Circulation 2017;136(3):314–26.

46. Sultan I, Kilic A, Kilic A. Short-term circulatory and right ventricle support in cardiogenic shock: extracorporeal membrane oxygenation, tandem heart, CentriMag, and Impella. Heart Fail Clin 2018; 14(4):579–83.

47. Schiller P, Vikholm P, Hellgren L. Experimental venoarterial extracorporeal membrane oxygenation induces left ventricular dysfunction. ASAIO J 2016;62(5):518–24.

48. Riebandt J, Haberl T, Wiedemann D, et al. Extracorporeal membrane oxygenation support for right

ventricular failure after left ventricular assist device implantation. Eur J Cardiothorac Surg 2018;53(3): 590–5.

49. Scherer M, Sirat AS, Moritz A, et al. Extracorporeal membrane oxygenation as perioperative right ventricular support in patients with biventricular failure undergoing left ventricular assist device implantation. Eur J Cardiothorac Surg 2011;39(6):939–44 [discussion: 944].

50. De Silva RJ, Soto C, Spratt P. Extra corporeal membrane oxygenation as right heart support following left ventricular assist device placement: a new cannulation technique. Heart Lung Circ 2012;21(4): 218–20.

51. Suguta M, Hoshizaki H, Anno M, et al. Right ventricular infarction with cardiogenic shock treated with percutaneous cardiopulmonary support: a case report. Jpn Circ J 1999;63(10):813–5.

52. Chopski SG, Murad NM, Fox CS, et al. Mechanical circulatory support of the right ventricle for adult and pediatric patients with heart failure. ASAIO J 2019;65(2):106–16.

53. Aggarwal V, Einhorn BN, Cohen HA. Current status of percutaneous right ventricular assist devices: first-in-man use of a novel dual lumen cannula. Catheter Cardiovasc Interv 2016;88(3):390–6.

54. Chung JS, Emerson D, Ramzy D, et al. A new paradigm in mechanical circulatory support: 100-patient experience. Ann Thorac Surg 2020; 109(5):1370–7.

55. Kapur NK, Paruchuri V, Korabathina R, et al. Effects of a percutaneous mechanical circulatory support device for medically refractory right ventricular failure. J Heart Lung Transplant 2011;30(12):1360–7.

56. Kapur NK, Paruchuri V, Jagannathan A, et al. Mechanical circulatory support for right ventricular failure. JACC Heart Fail 2013;1(2):127–34.

57. Ravichandran AK, Baran DA, Stelling K, et al. Outcomes with the tandem Protek duo dual-lumen percutaneous right ventricular assist device. ASAIO J 2018;64(4):570–2.

58. Bermundez CC SJ, Coletti AT, O'Neill BP, et al. Percutaneous right ventricular support: initial experience from the TandemHeart experiences and methods (THEME) registry. ASAIO J 2018;64:71.

59. Bermudez CA, Lagazzi L, Crespo MM. Prolonged support using a percutaneous OxyRVAD in a patient with end-stage lung disease, pulmonary hypertension, and right cardiac failure. ASAIO J 2016;62(4):e37–40.

60. Subramaniam K. Mechanical circulatory support. Best Pract Res Clin Anaesthesiol 2015;29(2):203–27.

61. Gregoric ID, Cohn WE, Akay MH, et al. CentriMag left ventricular assist system: cannulation through a right minithoracotomy. Tex Heart Inst J 2008;35(2): 184–5.

62. John R, Long JW, Massey HT, et al. Outcomes of a multicenter trial of the Levitronix CentriMag ventricular assist system for short-term circulatory support. J Thorac Cardiovasc Surg 2011;141(4):932–9.

63. Bhama JK, Kormos RL, Toyoda Y, et al. Clinical experience using the Levitronix CentriMag system for temporary right ventricular mechanical circulatory support. J Heart Lung Transplant 2009;28(9):971–6.

64. Mandawat A, Rao SV. Percutaneous mechanical circulatory support devices in cardiogenic shock. Circ Cardiovasc Interv 2017;10(5):e004337.

65. Ouweneel DM, Henriques JP. Percutaneous cardiac support devices for cardiogenic shock: current indications and recommendations. Heart 2012;98(16):1246–54.

66. Anderson MB, Goldstein J, Milano C, et al. Benefits of a novel percutaneous ventricular assist device for right heart failure: the prospective RECOVER RIGHT study of the Impella RP device. J Heart Lung Transplant 2015;34(12):1549–60.

67. Anderson M, Morris DL, Tang D, et al. Outcomes of patients with right ventricular failure requiring short-term hemodynamic support with the Impella RP device. J Heart Lung Transplant 2018;37(12):1448–58.

68. Bernhardt AM, De By TM, Reichenspurner H, et al. Isolated permanent right ventricular assist device implantation with the HeartWare continuous-flow ventricular assist device: first results from the European Registry for Patients with Mechanical Circulatory Support. Eur J Cardiothorac Surg 2015;48(1):158–62.

69. Shehab S, Macdonald PS, Keogh AM, et al. Long-term biventricular HeartWare ventricular assist device support–Case series of right atrial and right ventricular implantation outcomes. J Heart Lung Transplant 2016;35(4):466–73.

70. Lavee J, Mulzer J, Krabatsch T, et al. An international multicenter experience of biventricular support with HeartMate 3 ventricular assist systems. J Heart Lung Transplant 2018;37(12):1399–402.

71. Krabatsch T, Potapov E, Stepanenko A, et al. Biventricular circulatory support with two miniaturized implantable assist devices. Circulation 2011;124(11 Suppl):S179–86.

Extracorporeal Life Support and Mechanical Circulatory Support in Out-of-Hospital Cardiac Arrest and Refractory Cardiogenic Shock

Tyler M. Gunn, MD[a], Rajasekhar S.R. Malyala, MD[a],
John C. Gurley, MD[b],
Suresh Keshavamurthy, MD, FRCS[a],*

KEYWORDS

- Extracorporeal membrane oxygenation (ECMO) • Extracorporeal life support (ECLS)
- Extracorporeal cardiopulmonary resuscitation (ECPR) • Mechanical circulatory support (MCS)
- Out-of-hospital cardiac arrest (OHCA) • Refractory cardiogenic shock • Left ventricle unloading

---

KEY POINTS

- The prevalence of extracorporeal cardiopulmonary resuscitation is increasing worldwide as more health care centers develop the necessary infrastructure, protocols, and technical expertise.
- Early initiation of venoarterial (VA) extracorporeal life support (ECLS) in cases of refractory cardiogenic shock has been shown to improve survival and neurologic outcomes.
- Left ventricle unloading is an essential component of VA ECLS in the setting of cardiogenic shock and associated left ventricular dilation and is associated with improved survival and favorable outcomes.

BACKGROUND

Extracorporeal life support (ECLS) utilizes an extracorporeal membrane oxygenation (ECMO) circuit (**Fig. 1**), which comprises a venous outflow cannula, conduit tubing, blood pump (most commonly centrifugal), membrane lung (oxygenator), and inflow cannula inserted into either the venous or arterial system. In this article, the terms *outflow* (*efferent*) and *inflow* (*afferent*) refer to the direction of the blood flow relative to the patient, rather than the pump. Venovenous (VV) ECMO commonly is used in respiratory failure but rarely cardiogenic shock. Venoarterial (VA) ECMO is utilized in cardiogenic shock or cardiopulmonary arrest and involves venous

outflow to the circuit and return of oxygenated blood to the arterial circulation, replacing the majority of the function of the heart and lungs.

Extracorporeal cardiopulmonary resuscitation (ECPR) is the utilization of ECLS in situations of conventional cardiopulmonary resuscitation (CCPR) without successful return of spontaneous circulation (ROSC), or repetitive cardiac arrest after intermittent ROSC, as well as to facilitate interventions, such as coronary angiography, percutaneous catheter interventions, and operative procedures.[1] The development of smaller ECLS devices amenable to transportation, percutaneous cannulas allowing for rapid insertion, and cross-compatible extracorporeal

---

[a] Division of Cardiothoracic Surgery, University of Kentucky, 740 South Limestone, Suite A301, Lexington, KY 40536, USA; [b] Division of Cardiovascular Medicine, University of Kentucky, Gill Heart and Vascular Institute, 800 Rose Street, First Floor, Lexington, KY 40536, USA
* Corresponding author. Kentucky Clinic, 740 South Limestone, Suite A301, Lexington, KY 40536.
E-mail address: suresh.keshavamurthy@uky.edu

Intervent Cardiol Clin 10 (2021) 195–205
https://doi.org/10.1016/j.iccl.2020.12.006
2211-7458/21/© 2020 Elsevier Inc. All rights reserved.

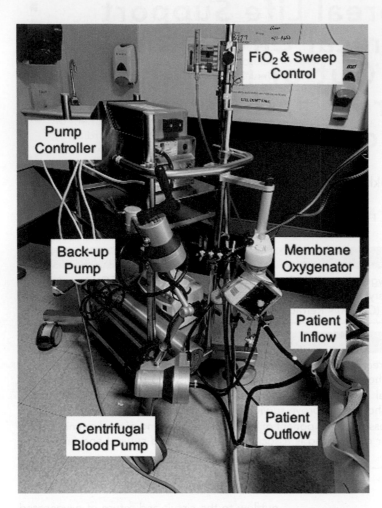

Fig. 1. VA ECMO circuit with centrifugal pump. FiO2, fraction of inspired oxygen.

FiO₂ & Sweep Control

Pump Controller

Back-up Pump

Membrane Oxygenator

Patient Inflow

Centrifugal Blood Pump

Patient Outflow

circuits has contributed to the technical feasibility and increasing popularity of ECPR. Definitions of refractory cardiac arrest vary but typically are considered 10 minutes to 30 minutes of CCPR without ROSC, but the optimal duration has not been determined for instances of both in-hospital cardiac arrest (IHCA) and out-of-hospital cardiac arrest (OHCA). Emergent percutaneous cannulation is performed in ECPR with the intent to provide full mechanical circulatory support (MCS) using a VA ECMO circuit. All patients with cardiac arrest may be eligible for ECPR; however, it is used more commonly in children and adults compared with neonates. This review focuses on the utilization of ECLS in the adult population. ECLS also may be indicated in situations of refractive cardiogenic shock, which is defined as systolic blood pressure less than 90 mm Hg, cardiac index less than 2.0 L/min/m², and evidence of end-organ hypoperfusion and multisystem organ failure despite aggressive pharmacologic interventions, including inotropes an vasopressors.[1] Other MCS devices may be indicated instead or concomitantly with the use of VA ECMO in refractory cardiogenic shock, including an intra-aortic balloon pump (IABP) and percutaneous or implantable univentricular assist device.

DISCUSSION
Prevalence and Trends of Extracorporeal Cardiopulmonary Resuscitation
Reports of percutaneous cardiopulmonary bypass for cardiac arrest or cardiogenic shock first were published more than a half century ago, and a systematic review of results in the literature between 1966 and 2005 reported a 42% survival to discharge.[2] Unfortunately, these exceptionally positive results likely were due to the historical under-reporting of poor outcomes. Leading regions in the development of ECPR initially comprised East Asia (including Japan), Republic of Korea, and Taiwan; trailed by

European countries, such as Germany, France, and Italy; and more recently the United States.[3] Utilization of ECLS for both OHCA and IHCA has become more prevalent in the United States over the past 2 decades. A study analyzing the National Inpatient Sample reported that between 2005 and 2014 the use of ECLS increased from 77 to 564 per 100,000 arrests for OHCA and from 60 to 632 per 100,000 arrests for IHCA, and the survival among patients on ECLS for OHCA and IHCA increased from 34.2% to 54.2% and from 4.7% to 19.2%, respectively.[4] ECPR remains a small fraction of the worldwide utilization of ECLS, with 9% (n = 6421) of 73,596 cases reported to the Extracorporeal Life Support Organization (ELSO) Registry as outlined in the January 2016 ELSO International Summary.[1]

Indications and Selection Criteria for Extracorporeal Cardiopulmonary Resuscitation in Out-of-Hospital Cardiac Arrest

ECPR is indicated in refractory cardiac arrest, which commonly is defined as 5 minutes to 30 minutes of CCPR without obtaining and sustaining ROSC. Selection criteria may include witnessed sudden arrest, assumption of cardiac etiology and reversible cause, high-quality CCPR initiated immediately after the cardiac arrest, achievement of intermittent ROSC, no major comorbidities or traditional contraindications to initiation of ECLS, and age under 70 years depending

---

> **Box 1**
> **Extracorporeal Life Support Organization patient selection criteria for extracorporeal cardiopulmonary resuscitation**
>
> Witnessed sudden arrest (catheter laboratory, operating room, intensive care unit, emergency department, public place, emergency medical service crew, and so forth)
>
> Immediate high-quality CPR with no sustained ROSC within 5 minutes to 15 minutes.
>
> Assumption of cardiac etiology and reversible cause (acute coronary syndrome, arrhythmia, myocarditis, pulmonary embolism).
>
> Intermittent ROSC
>
> No major comorbidities or ECLS contraindications (chronic organ dysfunction, terminal malignancy, prior CNS damage)
>
> Age under 70 years (case-by-case consideration based on functional status)

---

on patient functional status.[5,6] A compilation of the ELSO guidelines for ECPR patient selection criteria is outlined in **Box 1**.[1] Age limits for ECPR remain controversial and patients should be considered on a case-by-case basis. Potential organ donation is a consideration that has been used as an indication to proceed with ECPR.[1]

Outcomes for Extracorporeal Cardiopulmonary Resuscitation Compared with Conventional Cardiopulmonary Resuscitation

Primary outcomes measured in ECPR frequently include survival at hospital discharge or 30 days and favorable neurologic outcome. The rate of survival after ECPR in OHCA published in the literature ranges between 22% and 54%, with neurologically favorable survival between 4% and 29%.[1,7–9] An analysis of the ELSO registry between 2010 and 2016 by Haas and colleagues[8] reported that the survival to discharge of patients undergoing ECPR after OHCA worldwide was 28%, with brain death reported in 16.6% of patients.

Outcomes for ECPR have been compared with outcomes of CCPR in both IHCA and OHCA patient groups. In multiple recent studies, ECPR has demonstrated improved survival[9–12] and a better neurologic outcome[13] over CCPR in the setting of cardiac arrest. Chen and colleagues[10] published a 3-year prospective observational study of 172 patients in propensity score matched groups undergoing either ECPR or CCPR after IHCA and showed that ECPR significantly improved survival to discharge, 30-day survival, and 1-year survival. A systemic literature review and meta-analysis of 17 recent studies, performed by Twohig and colleagues,[9] found that ECPR demonstrated improved survival and better neurologic outcome over CCPR.

There is little consensus, however, in the literature regarding improved outcomes with ECPR. Two recently published large national registry reviews in France, by Bougouin and colleagues,[14] and in the Republic of Korea, by Choi and colleagues,[15] reported a statistically insignificant survival difference following ECPR compared with CCPR in OHCA. Patel and colleagues[16] reviewed the National Inpatient Sample between 2006 and 2014 in ECLS-capable facilities, which included 775 cases of ECPR after IHCA and reported a significantly higher mortality in patients who underwent ECPR than those who received CCPR and did not undergo ECPR. A systemic literature review of neurologic outcomes following ECPR in OHCA, performed by Beyea and colleagues,[17] found a trend toward improved survival and neurologic outcomes, but a preponderance of low-quality evidence may ascribe to optimism of a clinically relevant difference.

The inconsistency regarding published outcomes necessitates adequately powered randomized controlled trials to assess the benefit of ECPR in both OHCA and IHCA populations. The INCEPTION trial is a prospective multicenter trial enrolling in The Netherlands that aims to randomly allocate 110 patients to either ECPR or CCPR to explore survival and favorable neurologic outcomes; however, results have yet to be published.[18] An Australian study published in 2014 investigated refractory cardiac arrest treated with mechanical cardiopulmonary resuscitation (CPR), hypothermia, ECMO and early reperfusion (the CHEER trial) and reported favorable survival and neurologic outcome in 26 patients with either IHCA and OHCA.[19]

Differences in survival and neurologic outcome following ECPR between IHCA and OHCA patient populations have been investigated. OHCA patients typically are younger and have fewer medical comorbidities, and the cause of cardiac arrest more commonly is of cardiac origin; however, frequently they have longer low-flow times prior to initiation of ECLS. Review of recent studies indicates a higher rate of neurologically favorable survival in IHCA compared with OHCA patients.[1,20] More complex health care logistics as well as longer low-flow time may be a major contributing factor to worse outcomes in OHCA. A study 37 patients who underwent ECPR, published by Dennis and colleagues,[21] found comparable survival between IHCA (33%) and OHCA (37%) patient groups as well as favorable neurologic outcome in all survivors.

Predictors of Neurologic Outcomes After Extracorporeal Cardiopulmonary Resuscitation

Hypoxic ischemic brain injury remains a significant concern in ECPR after cardiac arrest and consists of a primary brain injury caused by the cessation of oxygen delivery as well as a secondary brain injury due to reperfusion following ROSC.[3] The main predictor of survival and neurologic function after cardiac arrest is time to treatment, and reduction of the low-flow time prior to initiation of ECPR is associated with favorable outcomes.[22–24] Wengenmayer and colleagues[22] reviewed 133 consecutive

patients who underwent ECPR for either IHCA or OHCA between 2010 and 2016 and found that low-flow time was shorter in IHCA than in OHCA patients, 49.6 minutes ± 5.9 minutes versus 72.2 minutes ± 7 minutes, respectively, and was correlated strongly with survival ($P<.0001$) and was an independent predictor of mortality. In another study, Otani and colleagues[23] published a review of 135 patients who underwent ECPR following OHCA between 2009 and 2017 and reported a statistically significant shorter median low-flow time in the favorable neurologic outcome group (38 minutes) compared with the unfavorable neurologic outcome group (48 minutes).

The American Heart Association (AHA) recommends the use of physical examination, such as the measurement of pupil diameter; imaging modalities, including computed tomography to assess gray matter–to–white matter ratio; electrophysiologic modalities, such as bispectral index and near-infrared spectroscopy; and laboratory examination of arterial blood gases and serum lactate to predict neurologic outcomes.[3,25] Utilization of a heat exchanger on the ECMO circuit provides the option of precise targeted temperature management (TTM) if indicated. The AHA recommends TTM between 32°C and 36°C after ROSC in patients with cardiac arrest, and TTM in the setting of ECPR has been associated with good neurologic outcomes.[23,26,27] The AHA recommends that prognostication of poor neurologic outcome should be delayed at least 72 hours after cardiac arrest or 72 hours after return to normothermia in patients treated with TTM.[25]

Complications of Extracorporeal Life Support

In addition to neurologic injury, there are many reported medical and procedural complications associated with ECLS. An analysis of the ELSO registry between 2010 and 2016 reported complications, including cardiovascular complications (53.0%), renal failure (27.7%), neurologic complications (24.0%), hemorrhage (31.3%), limb ischemia or vascular injury (11.1%), ECMO circuit complications (8.8%), and infection (7.4%), while both neurologic and infectious complications were the only statistically significant contributors to mortality.[8] Major bleeding is the most common procedural complication, with an estimated prevalence of 30% to 42% in ECLS patients, of which 25% to 63% require operative management.[1,28] Common locations of bleeding include cannulation sites and gastrointestinal tract and less commonly central nervous system and pulmonary hemorrhage, as well as bleeding from disseminated intravascular coagulation. Lower extremity arterial cannulation predisposes patients to limb ischemia, frequently requiring fasciotomy and possible amputation, and often necessitates the placement of small distal reperfusion catheter. Appropriate and proactive management of postprocedural complications has a significant impact on ECLS patient outcomes.

Extracorporeal Life Support and Temporary Mechanical Circulatory Support in Refractory Cardiogenic Shock

Cardiogenic shock commonly is defined as decreased cardiac output resulting in tissue hypoxia in the presence of adequate intravascular volume. This may be subsequent to left, right, or biventricular failure. Acute coronary syndrome is the most common cause of cardiogenic shock and represents approximately 70% to 80% of cases.[29-31] Other causes of cardiogenic shock include decompensation of chronic heart failure and right heart failure; postcardiotomy, viral, autoimmune, or stress cardiomyopathy; hypertrophic cardiomyopathy; myocarditis; acute valvular disease; endocarditis; cardiac contusion; and sustained arrythmias.[32] Postcardiotomy cardiogenic shock may develop in 2% to 6% of patients undergoing cardiac surgery.[31,33] The use of temporary MCS has become more prevalent than durable left ventricular (LV) assist devices because they are less invasive, less complicated to insert in critically ill patients, and less expensive.

The Society for Cardiovascular Angiography and Interventions (SCAI) has developed a classification of cardiogenic shock that incorporates physical examination, biochemical markers, and hemodynamics and ranges from A to E, with stage A "at risk" for cardiogenic shock, stage B is "beginning" shock, stage C "classic" cardiogenic shock, stage D "deteriorating," and stage E "extremis."[34] Widely accepted indications, selection criteria, and optimal timing for initiation of temporary MCS ahve not yet been determined. It is estimated that only 15% to 25% of patients with cardiogenic shock may be appropriate for temporary MCS, considering that approximately 50% to 60% of patients survive with medical therapy, and in another 25% to 35% of patients temporary MCS may be futile due to irreversible organ failure and anoxic brain injury.[30,35] Jentzer and colleagues[36] reviewed more than 10,000 patients with cardiogenic shock admitted to the Mayo Clinic between 2007 and 2015 and reported the frequency rates of patients with SCAI stages A through E were

46.0%, 30.0%, 15.7%, 7.3%, and 1.0%, respectively; and unadjusted hospital mortality rates in these stages were 3.0%, 7.1%, 12.4%, 40.4%, and 67.0%, respectively. Varying strategies and techniques complicate predicted survival in ECLS for refractory cardiogenic shock but are estimated to be approximately 40%.[37-39] Early escalation of temporary MCS, including VA ECLS and LV unloading, has been shown to enable stabilization and may rescue high-risk patients with refractory cardiogenic shock at low overall risk.[37]

TECHNIQUES

Extracorporeal Life Support Techniques in Extracorporeal Cardiopulmonary Resuscitation Refractory Cardiogenic Shock

VA ECMO is utilized in ECPR and refractory cardiogenic shock and involves venous outflow to the circuit and return of oxygenated blood to the arterial circulation, replacing the majority of the function of the heart and lungs. In emergent situations, such as in both IHCA and OHCA, femoral arterial and femoral venous cannulation is preferred. Cannulation of the common femoral artery is preferred because of its larger diameter and decreased risk of distal limb ischemia and vessel injury. Appropriately large cannulas should be selected in the setting of ECPR and ECLS for refractory cardiogenic shock to allow for full flows to temporally replace cardiac output, typically 15F to 18F arterial cannulas. Distal limb ischemia and bleeding, especially after therapeutic anticoagulation, are significant complications that have an impact on patient survival. A distal reperfusion catheter (typically 5F–7F) may be inserted into the superficial femoral artery under ultrasound guidance and be attached directly to the EMCO inflow circuit, which provides improved distal limb perfusion.

The right femoral vein is the preferred venous cannulation site because of a straighter course proximally towards the common iliac vein and the inferior vena cava. A portable chest and abdominal radiogram should be obtained to verify arterial and venous cannula positioning. Cannulas must be well secured in multiple locations, especially the arterial cannula due to its small size and length; a purse-string suture at the insertion site is commonly placed and may decrease bleeding once therapeutic anticoagulation is initiated.

If femoral artery cannulation is unsuccessful bilaterally or aborted due to known peripheral vascular disease or observed calcification, emergent cannulation of the left axillary artery is a potential alternative. The left axillary artery is preferred to the right due to its direct anatomic path to the aortic arch, whereas the right axillary artery involves the right carotid artery via the brachiocephalic artery and may increase the incidence of stroke. When percutaneous cannulation is not successful and when it is undesirable to interrupt CPR, an emergent groin cutdown to access femoral artery and vein is helpful to institute ECLS. The axillary artery is more difficult to access, of smaller diameter, and more prone to vessel wall injury than the femoral artery. A smaller 15F arterial cannula typically is placed in the axillary artery, providing enough flow to the ascending aorta while minimizing vessel trauma and risk of distal limb ischemia but may require surgical repositioning at a later time.

Nonemergent and Open Surgical Extracorporeal Life Support Cannulation Technique

Nonemergent scenarios of refractory cardiogenic shock allow for better assessment of vascular anatomy and pathology and for planning of techniques that decrease the risk of complications. Open surgical peripheral cannulation techniques include right or left axillary artery exploration with anastomosis of a Dacron graft extension, which can be connected directly to the ECMO inflow tubing or house an arterial cannula. When patients improve, surgical decannulation may be simplified by the stapling of the graft just distal to the anastomosis and not require axillary artery repair. When compared with other peripheral cannulation techniques, open axillary cannulation likely decreases the risk of limb ischemia and insufficient arterial mixing of native deoxygenated arterial blood and oxygenated blood from the peripheral inflow cannula. Harlequin syndrome in the setting of femoral VA ECLS, sometimes referred to as north-south syndrome, results from distal migration into the ascending, transverse, or descending thoracic aorta of the mixing cloud between the native deoxygenated arterial blood ejected from the LV and oxygenated blood from the peripheral inflow cannula. This results in insufficiently oxygenated arterial blood flow to the coronary arteries, head, brain, and upper extremities.

Central (surgical) arterial cannulation may be indicated in patients with postcardiotomy cardiogenic shock, postoperative patients with recent sternotomy, and patients on peripheral VA ECLS with distal limb ischemia or harlequin syndrome. Central cannulation involves direct arterial cannulation of the ascending aorta and either cannulation of the right atrial appendage or peripheral venous cannulation of the femoral vein. Central cannulation frequently is associated with mediastinal bleeding requiring increased blood transfusion and surgical exploration, and peripheral cannulation commonly is associated with increased limb ischemia and vascular injury.[40–42] Raffa and colleagues[42] performed a meta-analysis of 17 retrospective studies containing 1691 patients with postcardiotomy and non-postcardiotomy cardiogenic shock who underwent central or peripheral cannulation and reported comparable in-hospital survival between central and peripheral cannulation, although the risk of bleeding, continuous VV hemofiltration, and blood product transfusion was significantly lower with peripheral cannulation.

Left Ventricle Unloading Strategies

ECMO flow should be high enough for sufficient replacement of cardiac output but allow for some blood flow through the right heart, lungs, and left heart to avoid venous stasis and thrombosis. Adequate hemodynamics and organ perfusion should be obtained with a target mean arterial pressure above 65 mm Hg and mixed venous oxygen saturation greater than 55%. Ventricular ejections can be monitored on arterial line tracings and bedside (pulse pressure >10 mm Hg) transthoracic echocardiography, with special attention to observe LV decompression and aortic valve opening, especially in the presence of a mechanical prosthesis, which is prone to thrombosis. If a Swan-Ganz catheter is placed, both increased pulmonary artery diastolic pressure (>25 mm Hg) and elevated pulmonary capillary wedge pressure are evidence of LV distension.[43] VA ECLS generates increased afterload in the aorta, which interferes with ejections from the diminished LV, which may lead to distension and potential intracardiac thrombus formation. LV distension leads to amplified LV wall stress and increased oxygen demands, and elevated LV end-diastolic pressure results in subendocardial ischemia, which eventually may lead to the development of ventricular arrhythmias.[44] A form of LV unloading is indicated if LV distension is observed or suspected in the setting of VA ECLS, and multiple studies have indicated increased survival with early LV decompression.[45–47] A meta-analysis of 3997 patients with refractory cardiogenic shock on VA ECLS, including 1696 patients with concomitant LV unloading, reported a significant mortality reduction with LV unloading.[45] Another large meta-analysis, published by Al-Fares and colleagues,[46] found an increased success of VA ECLS weaning and reduced short-term mortality with LV unloading, especially if performed early (<12 hours).

Techniques to offload the LV include conservative medical management and concomitant surgical venting or separate invasive procedures and device placement. Medical management involves the use of inotropes, such as milrinone, dopamine, and dobutamine, which increase LV contractility and contribute modestly to cardiac output. Aggressive diuresis and the use of continuous VV hemofiltration can decrease volume overload while conservative doses of vasopressors maintain blood pressure.[48] An IABP is a percutaneous option to aid in LV decompression and works by augmenting coronary artery blood flow and decreasing aortic afterload but does not directly vent the LV. The benefit of IABP in LV unloading in the setting of VA ECLS, however, is controversial and a pooled study of 1517 patients, published by Cheng and colleagues,[49,50] found that there was no significant survival benefit associated with concomitant IABP placement.

Percutaneous left atrial vents and the TandemHeart system (LivaNova, London, England) provide left atrial drainage via a transseptal puncture under fluoroscopic guidance. Percutaneous vents include transseptal puncture and left atrial drain placement, transseptal balloon septostomy, and percutaneous insertion of a pulmonary artery vent. Left atrial VA ECLS is a technique involving a percutaneous transseptal puncture with tip insertion of the femoral venous cannula into the left atrium under fluoroscopic guidance and can be performed with initial cannulation or as a modification to preexisting VA ECLS with femoral venous outflow cannula replacement (Fig. 2). This provides LV offloading via the left atrium while maintaining venous cannula outflow sufficient for full cardiac output replacement. Percutaneous pulmonary artery venting is another minimally invasive approach that has been described to indirectly unload the LV with some success, although this technique has not gained widespread acceptance.[51]

The Impella device (Abiomed, Danvers, Massachusetts) is another percutaneous LV unloading option. In VA ECLS, the majority of the cardiac output already is being replaced by the ECMO circuit, and a smaller Impella CP can adequately decompress the LV, with an expected flow of 1.5 L/min to 2.0 L/min, which sometimes is referred to as ECPELLA (Fig. 3). During weaning from ECLS, the Impella CP® flow is maintained and often left after ECLS decannulation to augment cardiac output if required prior to removal. Pappalardo and colleagues[52] published a review of 157 patients placed on either VA ECLS alone or VA ECLS with an Impella and found that patients with LV decompression with Impella had a significantly lower mortality and a higher rate of successful bridging to either recovery or further therapy. In a comparison of 45 patients on VA ECLS at Washington University, who concomitantly received either a surgical LV vent or an Impella, Tepper and colleagues[53] reported that pulmonary artery diastolic pressure and radiographic evidence of pulmonary edema were reduced significantly in the Impella group; however, differences in survival were not statistically significant. A meta-analysis of 8 studies reporting LV unloading during VA ECLS, performed by Meuwese and colleagues,[54] reported that LV unloading was associated with a significant reduction in LV preload parameters, and the effect was most pronounced in Impella and atrial septostomy groups. The use of an Impella as stand-alone temporary MCS after myocardial infarction and percutaneous coronary intervention has garnered recent controversy due to concerns regarding efficacy and resource stewardship

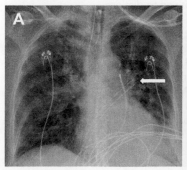 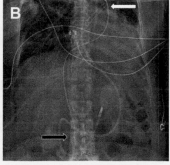

Fig. 2. (A) Chest radiograph with left atrial VA ECLS with transseptal puncture with femoral venous outflow cannula tip into the left atrium (arrow) and (B) abdominal radiograph showing both venous outflow cannula in the left atrium (white arrow) and femoral arterial inflow cannula tip (black arrow). (Courtesy of the University of Kentucky IRB, Lexington, KY; with permission.)

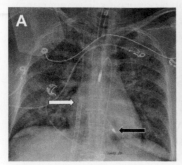 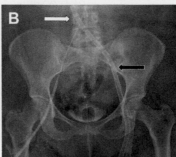

Fig. 3. (*A*) Chest radiograph with femoral venous outflow cannula tip at the right atrial and superior vena cava confluence (*white arrow*) with Impella CP placement across the aortic valve into the LV (*black arrow*) and (*B*) pelvic radiograph showing both venous outflow cannula (*white arrow*) and shorter femoral arterial inflow cannula tip (*black arrow*). (*Courtesy of* the University of Kentucky IRB, Lexington, KY; with permission.)

after analysis of the IABP-SHOCK II trial showed Impella was not associated with lower 30-day mortality compared with IABP,[55] and a large review published in 2019 revealed that Impella use was associated with higher rates of adverse events and costs.[56]

Surgical options for LV unloading in postcardiotomy cardiogenic shock include the placement of a left pulmonary vein cannula, which is connected into the venous outflow back to the ECMO circuit but unfortunately is prone to thrombosis. Another technique involving LV unloading if through the use of a CentriMag (Abbott, Chicago, Illinois) ventricular assist device integrated with VA ECLS, which was developed at Columbia University and comprises drainage from the apex of the LV, which is combined with venous outflow from the jugular or femoral vein; the arterial inflow is returned to the axillary artery or ascending aorta through a hemisternotomy.[43] Benefits of this approach include perfusing oxygenated blood antegrade from the upper body, unloading the right ventricle and LV efficiently, potential to ambulate the patient by removing venous ECLS limb, and potential to avoid reoperative sternotomy for subsequent durable LV assist device placement or heart transplant.[43]

SUMMARY

The prevalence of ECPR is increasing worldwide as more health care centers develop the necessary infrastructure, protocols, and technical expertise required to provide mobile ECLS with short notice. Strict adherence to patient selection guidelines in the setting of OHCA allows for improved survival with neurologically favorable outcomes in a larger patient population. Technical advances in VA ECLS and temporary MCS, with an emphasis on LV unloading, have increased survival in refractory cardiogenic shock.

CLINICS CARE POINTS

- Selection criteria for ECPR include witnessed sudden arrest, assumption of cardiac etiology and reversible cause, high-quality CCPR initiated immediately after the cardiac arrest, achievement of intermittent ROSC, no major comorbidities or traditional contraindications to initiation of ECLS, and age under 70 years depending on patient functional status.

- The main predictor of survival and satisfactory neurologic function is the reduction of low-flow time prior to initiation of ECPR.

- Early initiation of VA ECLS in the setting of refractory cardiogenic shock has been shown to improve survival and neurologic outcomes.

- LV unloading is critical in the setting of cardiogenic shock and LV dilation and commonly is accomplished by Impella placement, IABP, transseptal puncture, or pulmonary artery venting.

DISCLOSURE

Authors have nothing to disclose.

REFERENCES

1. Brogan TV, Lequier L, Lorusso R, et al. Extracorporeal life support: the ELSO red book. 5th edition. Ann Arbor (MI): Extracorporeal Life Support Organization; 2017.

2. Nichol G, Karmy-Jones R, Salerno C, et al. Systematic review of percutaneous cardiopulmonary bypass for cardiac arrest or cardiogenic shock states. Resuscitation 2006;70(3):381–94.

3. Inoue A, Hifumi T, Sakamoto T, et al. Extracorporeal cardiopulmonary resuscitation for out-of-hospital cardiac arrest in adult patients. J Am Heart Assoc 2020;9(7):e015291.

4. Hadaya J, Dobaria V, Aguayo E, et al. National trends in utilization and outcomes of extracorporeal support for in- and out-of-hospital cardiac arrest. Resuscitation 2020;151:181–8.

5. Reynolds JC, Frisch A, Rittenberger JC, et al. Duration of resuscitation efforts and functional outcome after out-of-hospital cardiac arrest: when should we change to novel therapies? Circulation 2013; 128(23):2488–94.

6. Bossaert LL, Perkins GD, Askitopoulou H, et al. European resuscitation council guidelines for resuscitation 2015: Section 11. The ethics of resuscitation and end-of-life decisions. Resuscitation 2015;95: 302–11.

7. Ortega-Deballon I, Hornby L, Shemie SD, et al. Extracorporeal resuscitation for refractory out-of-hospital cardiac arrest in adults: a systematic review of international practices and outcomes. Resuscitation 2016;101:12–20.

8. Haas NL, Coute RA, Hsu CH, et al. Descriptive analysis of extracorporeal cardiopulmonary resuscitation following out-of-hospital cardiac arrest-An ELSO registry study. Resuscitation 2017;119:56–62.

9. Twohig CJ, Singer B, Grier G, et al. A systematic literature review and meta-analysis of the effectiveness of extracorporeal-CPR versus conventional-CPR for adult patients in cardiac arrest. J Intensive Care Soc 2019;20(4):347–57.

10. Chen YS, Lin JW, Yu HY, et al. Cardiopulmonary resuscitation with assisted extracorporeal life-support versus conventional cardiopulmonary resuscitation in adults with in-hospital cardiac arrest: an observational study and propensity analysis. Lancet 2008;372(9638):554–61.

11. Pozzi M, Armoiry X, Achana F, et al. Extracorporeal life support for refractory cardiac arrest: a 10-year comparative analysis. Ann Thorac Surg 2019; 107(3):809–16.

12. Sun T, Guy A, Sidhu A, et al. Veno-arterial extracorporeal membrane oxygenation (VA-ECMO) for emergency cardiac support. J Crit Care 2018;44: 31–8.

13. Sakamoto T, Morimura N, Nagao K, et al. Extracorporeal cardiopulmonary resuscitation versus conventional cardiopulmonary resuscitation in adults with out-of-hospital cardiac arrest: a prospective observational study. Resuscitation 2014;85(6):762–8.

14. Bougouin W, Dumas F, Lamhaut L, et al. Extracorporeal cardiopulmonary resuscitation in out-of-hospital cardiac arrest: a registry study. Eur Heart J 2020;41(21):1961–71.

15. Choi DS, Kim T, Ro YS, et al. Extracorporeal life support and survival after out-of-hospital cardiac arrest in a nationwide registry: a propensity score-matched analysis. Resuscitation 2016;99:26–32.

16. Patel JK, Meng H, Qadeer A, et al. Impact of extracorporeal membrane oxygenation on mortality in adults with cardiac arrest. Am J Cardiol 2019; 124(12):1857–61.

17. Beyea MM, Tillmann BW, Iansavichene AE, et al. Neurologic outcomes after extracorporeal membrane oxygenation assisted CPR for resuscitation of out-of-hospital cardiac arrest patients: a systematic review. Resuscitation 2018;130:146–58.

18. Bol ME, Suverein MM, Lorusso R, et al. Early initiation of extracorporeal life support in refractory out-of-hospital cardiac arrest: Design and rationale of the INCEPTION trial. Am Heart J 2019;210:58–68.

19. Stub D, Bernard S, Pellegrino V, et al. Refractory cardiac arrest treated with mechanical CPR, hypothermia, ECMO and early reperfusion (the CHEER trial). Resuscitation 2015;86:88–94.

20. Lunz D, Calabro L, Belliato M, et al. Extracorporeal membrane oxygenation for refractory cardiac arrest: a retrospective multicenter study. Intensive Care Med 2020;46(5):973–82.

21. Dennis M, McCanny P, D'Souza M, et al. Extracorporeal cardiopulmonary resuscitation for refractory cardiac arrest: a multicentre experience. Int J Cardiol 2017;231:131–6.

22. Wengenmayer T, Rombach S, Ramshorn F, et al. Influence of low-flow time on survival after extracorporeal cardiopulmonary resuscitation (eCPR). Crit Care 2017;21(1):157.

23. Otani T, Sawano H, Natsukawa T, et al. Low-flow time is associated with a favorable neurological outcome in out-of-hospital cardiac arrest patients resuscitated with extracorporeal cardiopulmonary resuscitation. J Crit Care 2018;48:15–20.

24. Leick J, Liebetrau C, Szardien S, et al. Door-to-implantation time of extracorporeal life support systems predicts mortality in patients with out-of-hospital cardiac arrest. Clin Res Cardiol 2013; 102(9):661–9.

25. Callaway CW, Donnino MW, Fink EL, et al. Part 8: post-cardiac arrest care: 2015 American heart association guidelines update for cardiopulmonary resuscitation and emergency cardiovascular care. Circulation 2015;132(18 Suppl 2):S465–82.

26. Kim SJ, Jung JS, Park JH, et al. An optimal transition time to extracorporeal cardiopulmonary resuscitation for predicting good neurological outcome in patients with out-of-hospital cardiac arrest: a propensity-matched study. Crit Care 2014;18(5):535.

27. Nagao K, Kikushima K, Watanabe K, et al. Early induction of hypothermia during cardiac arrest improves neurological outcomes in patients with out-of-hospital cardiac arrest who undergo emergency cardiopulmonary bypass and percutaneous coronary intervention. Circ J 2010;74(1):77–85.

28. Mazzeffi M, Greenwood J, Tanaka K, et al. Bleeding, transfusion, and mortality on extracorporeal life support: ECLS working group on thrombosis and hemostasis. Ann Thorac Surg 2016; 101(2):682–9.

29. Harjola VP, Lassus J, Sionis A, et al. Clinical picture and risk prediction of short-term mortality in cardiogenic shock. Eur J Heart Fail 2015;17(5): 501–9.

30. Combes A, Price S, Slutsky AS, et al. Temporary circulatory support for cardiogenic shock. Lancet 2020;396(10245):199–212.

31. van Diepen S, Katz JN, Albert NM, et al. Contemporary management of cardiogenic shock: a scientific statement from the american heart association. Circulation 2017;136(16):e232–68.

32. Wilcox SR. Nonischemic causes of cardiogenic shock. Emerg Med Clin North Am 2019;37(3): 493–509.

33. Mohite PN, Sabashnikov A, Patil NP, et al. Short-term ventricular assist device in post-cardiotomy cardiogenic shock: factors influencing survival. J Artif Organs 2014;17(3):228–35.

34. Baran DA, Grines CL, Bailey S, et al. SCAI clinical expert consensus statement on the classification of cardiogenic shock: this document was endorsed by the American college of cardiology (ACC), the American heart association (AHA), the society of critical care medicine (SCCM), and the society of thoracic surgeons (STS) in April 2019. Catheter Cardiovasc Interv 2019;94(1):29–37.

35. Thiele H, Ohman EM, de Waha-Thiele S, et al. Management of cardiogenic shock complicating myocardial infarction: an update 2019. Eur Heart J 2019;40(32):2671–83.

36. Jentzer JC, van Diepen S, Barsness GW, et al. Cardiogenic shock classification to predict mortality in the cardiac intensive care unit. J Am Coll Cardiol 2019;74(17):2117–28.

37. Tongers J, Sieweke JT, Kuhn C, et al. Early escalation of mechanical circulatory support stabilizes and potentially rescues patients in refractory cardiogenic shock. Circ Heart Fail 2020;13(3):e005853.

38. Thiagarajan RR, Barbaro RP, Rycus PT, et al. Extracorporeal life support organization registry international report 2016. ASAIO J 2017;63(1):60–7.

39. Combes A, Leprince P, Luyt CE, et al. Outcomes and long-term quality-of-life of patients supported by extracorporeal membrane oxygenation for refractory cardiogenic shock. Crit Care Med 2008; 36(5):1404–11.

40. Djordjevic I, Eghbalzadeh K, Sabashnikov A, et al. Central vs peripheral venoarterial ECMO in postcardiotomy cardiogenic shock. J Cardiovasc Surg 2020;35(5):1037–42.

41. Ranney DN, Benrashid E, Meza JM, et al. Central cannulation as a viable alternative to peripheral cannulation in extracorporeal membrane oxygenation. Semin Thorac Cardiovasc Surg 2017;29(2): 188–95.

42. Raffa GM, Kowalewski M, Brodie D, et al. Meta-analysis of peripheral or central extracorporeal membrane oxygenation in postcardiotomy and non-postcardiotomy shock. Ann Thorac Surg 2019;107(1):311–21.

43. Cevasco M, Takayama H, Ando M, et al. Left ventricular distension and venting strategies for patients on venoarterial extracorporeal membrane oxygenation. J Thorac Dis 2019; 11(4):1676–83.

44. Burkhoff D, Sayer G, Doshi D, et al. Hemodynamics of mechanical circulatory support. J Am Coll Cardiol 2015;66(23):2663–74.

45. Russo JJ, Aleksova N, Pitcher I, et al. Left ventricular unloading during extracorporeal membrane oxygenation in patients with cardiogenic shock. J Am Coll Cardiol 2019;73(6):654–62.

46. Al-Fares AA, Randhawa VK, Englesakis M, et al. Optimal strategy and timing of left ventricular venting during veno-arterial extracorporeal life support for adults in cardiogenic shock: a systematic review and meta-analysis. Circ Heart Fail 2019;12(11): e006486.

47. Pineton de Chambrun M, Brechot N, Combes A. The place of extracorporeal life support in cardiogenic shock. Curr Opin Crit Care 2020;26(4): 424–31.

48. Touchan J, Guglin M. Temporary mechanical circulatory support for cardiogenic shock. Curr Treat Options Cardiovasc Med 2017;19(10):77.

49. Cheng R, Hachamovitch R, Makkar R, et al. Lack of survival benefit found with use of intraaortic balloon pump in extracorporeal membrane oxygenation: a pooled experience of 1517 patients. J Invasive Cardiol 2015;27(10):453–8.

50. Nagpal AD, Singal RK, Arora RC, et al. Temporary mechanical circulatory support in cardiac critical care: a state of the art review and algorithm for device selection. Can J Cardiol 2017; 33(1):110–8.

51. Avalli L, Maggioni E, Sangalli F, et al. Percutaneous left-heart decompression during extracorporeal membrane oxygenation: an alternative to surgical and transeptal venting in adult patients. ASAIO J 2011;57(1):38–40.

52. Pappalardo F, Schulte C, Pieri M, et al. Concomitant implantation of Impella((R)) on top of veno-arterial extracorporeal membrane oxygenation may improve survival of patients with cardiogenic shock. Eur J Heart Fail 2017;19(3):404–12.

53. Tepper S, Masood MF, Baltazar Garcia M, et al. Left Ventricular Unloading by Impella Device Versus Surgical Vent During Extracorporeal Life Support. Ann Thorac Surg 2017;104(3):861–7.

54. Meuwese CL, de Haan M, Zwetsloot PP, et al. The hemodynamic effect of different left ventricular unloading techniques during veno-arterial extracorporeal life support: a systematic review and meta-analysis. Perfusion 2020;35. 267659119897478.

55. Schrage B, Ibrahim K, Loehn T, et al. Impella support for acute myocardial infarction complicated by cardiogenic shock. Circulation 2019;139(10): 1249–58.

56. Amin AP, Spertus JA, Curtis JP, et al. The evolving landscape of impella use in the united states among patients undergoing percutaneous coronary intervention with mechanical circulatory support. Circulation 2020;141(4):273–84.

Mechanical Circulatory Support in High-Risk Percutaneous Coronary Intervention

Katherine J. Kunkel, MD, MSEd[a],*,
Mohammed Ferras Dabbagh, MD[b],
Mohammad Zaidan, MD[a], Khaldoon Alaswad, MD[a]

KEYWORDS

- High-risk percutaneous coronary intervention • Mechanical circulatory support
- Coronary artery disease • Risk assessment • Hemodynamics
- Percutaneous coronary intervention • Heart-assist devices

KEY POINTS

- Identifying patients at high risk for percutaneous coronary intervention (PCI) involves a synthesis of a patient comorbidities, hemodynamic status, and lesion characteristics.
- Mechanical circulatory support devices are used in high-risk PCI to augment cardiac output and reduce myocardial oxygen demand during coronary intervention.
- The use of mechanical circulatory support devices allows more complete revascularization and facilitates procedures that previously may not have been technically feasible.
- Prospective randomized trials to date have not shown a benefit for the routine use of mechanical circulatory support in patients with low ejection fraction and a high burden of coronary disease.
- Further research is required to identify groups that will receive the maximal benefit of mechanical circulatory support in high-risk PCI.

INTRODUCTION

Coronary artery disease remains a leading worldwide cause of morbidity and mortality.[1] As medical and interventional therapies available to patients with atherosclerotic heart disease have improved, the number of patients surviving index coronary events has increased considerably.[2] The care of this older, more medically and anatomically complex group of patients has resulted in an increasing number of patients with indications for coronary revascularization who are at high risk of periprocedural hemodynamic collapse and increased morbidity and mortality.[3]

Concurrently, the technology available to perform complex percutaneous coronary interventions (PCIs) has dramatically improved with the advent of coronary guides and guide extensions, specialized coronary wires, atherectomy devices, lower profile balloons and stents, intravascular imaging, specialized equipment for chronic total occlusions (CTOs), and percutaneous mechanical circulatory support (MCS) devices.[4] Patients who previously may not have been offered coronary revascularization because of technical factors or risk associated with cardiac surgery can now be considered for percutaneous revascularization. A clinical case that exemplifies this patient population is

[a] Interventional Cardiology, Henry Ford Hospital, 2799 West Grand Boulevard, K-2, Detroit, MI 48202, USA;
[b] Division of Cardiology, Henry Ford Hospital, 2799 West Grand Boulevard, K-14, Detroit, MI 48202, USA
* Corresponding author.
E-mail address: kkunkel2@hfhs.org

Intervent Cardiol Clin 10 (2021) 207–219
https://doi.org/10.1016/j.iccl.2020.12.002
2211-7458/21/© 2020 Elsevier Inc. All rights reserved.

a 66-year-old man with a history of alcohol abuse who presented to an outside facility with 1 hour of chest pain. He rapidly developed hypoxic respiratory failure, and intubation was complicated by polymorphic ventricular tachycardia and cardiac arrest. Urgent cardiac catheterization was notable for cardiogenic shock with a cardiac index of 0.9 L/min/m^2 and severe 3-vessel coronary artery disease, with CTOs of the right and left circumflex coronary arteries and a highly calcific 95% stenosis of the proximal left anterior descending coronary artery (Fig. 1). The patient was urgently transferred to a tertiary referral center where, given severe peripheral arterial disease and cardiogenic shock, a transcaval Impella 5.0 was placed (Fig. 2). After stabilization of end-organ function, the patient underwent successful atherectomy and PCI of the left main to left anterior descending (LAD) artery (Fig. 3). The patient ultimately was successfully weaned from MCS and discharged to rehabilitation in good condition. In patients such as this and many others with high-risk lesions and clinical risk, a key element that has facilitated PCI is the advent of percutaneous MCS.

Percutaneous MCS in PCI is generally used in one of 2 clinical settings: patients with acute myocardial infarctions (MIs) presenting with cardiogenic shock, and patients electively undergoing planned high-risk PCI.[5] In this article, the use of MCS in elective high-risk PCI is discussed.

Although the use of MCS in high-risk PCI has been theorized to allow safer, more complete coronary interventions, MCS in high-risk PCI has not conclusively been shown to be associated with improved clinical outcomes in prospective randomized clinical trials.[6,7] This article discusses the elements of decision making in the use of hemodynamic support in high-risk PCI, the current state of the evidence base for the use of MCS in high-risk PCI, and a practical approach to clinical decision making.

DEFINING HIGH-RISK PERCUTANEOUS CORONARY INTERVENTION

At present, there is no standardized definition of high-risk PCI. Although risk calculators exist for both coronary artery bypass grafting (CABG) and PCI,[8,9] experts believe that these calculators do not adequately capture the complexity of this patient group.[10,11]

All proposed definitions of high-risk PCI incorporate 3 general categories of factors that, in combination, designate a procedure as high risk and can justify the use of periprocedural MCS: patient-specific comorbidities,

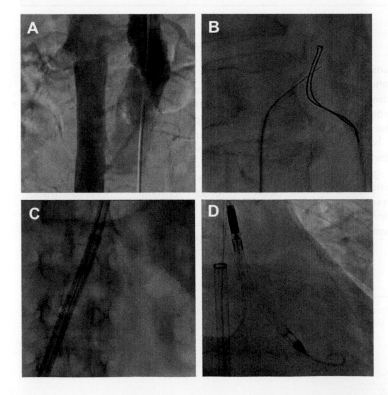

Fig. 1. Transcaval insertion of an intravascular micro-axial pump delivering up to 5.0 L/min with (A) simultaneous IVC and aorta angiography, (B) transcaval puncture, (C) 24 French sheath advancement, and (D) device positioning.

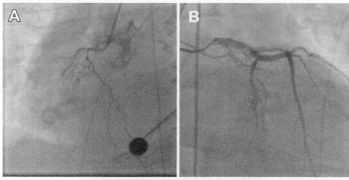

Fig. 2. Diagnostic angiography showing (A) a CTO of the right coronary artery as well as a CTO of the left circumflex and an eccentric, calcific stenosis of the proximal left anterior descending coronary artery (B, C).

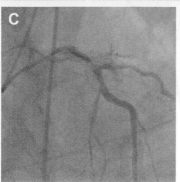

hemodynamic factors, and factors specific to lesion and procedural technique (Fig. 4).[5,12] The relative importance of each of these factors in this qualitative assessment of procedural risk

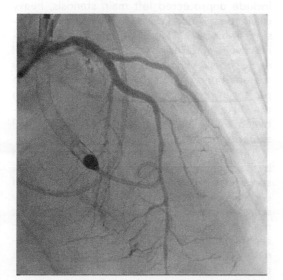

Fig. 3. Completion angiogram following intravascular micro-axial pump supported atherectomy of the proximal left anterior descending coronary artery and bifurcation stenting with the first diagonal branch.

is unknown and remains a future direction for research.

Patient-Specific Factors

Comorbid diabetes mellitus, chronic lung disease, chronic kidney disease, prior MI, reduced left ventricular ejection fraction (LVEF), and peripheral arterial disease have all been associated with worse outcomes in PCI.[13–17] Advanced age and frailty are also associated with higher morbidity and mortality in patients undergoing PCI.[18] The aggregate of the patient's underlying health status is an important factor in determining the patient's ability to tolerate the stresses of transient ischemia, bleeding, arrhythmias, and hypotension often encountered in high-risk PCI. Patients with a lower physiologic reserve are more likely to incur end-organ dysfunction and ultimately mortality as a result of the hemodynamic stress of PCI and should be more strongly considered for the use of MCS.

Hemodynamic Status

The acuity of the clinical presentation before PCI remains the strongest predictor of procedural major adverse events.[19] PCI in the setting of acute coronary syndrome confers a higher risk of adverse events than elective PCI. Symptomatic heart failure with increased filling pressures

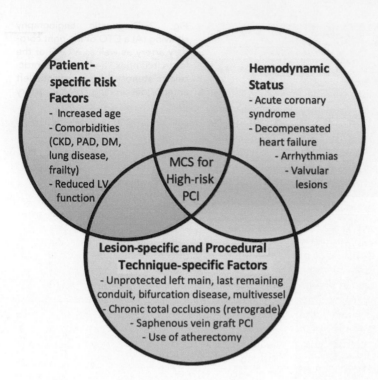

Fig. 4. Contributing factors in defining the high-risk PCI patient group most likely to benefit from invasive hemodynamic assessment and the use of MCS. CKD, chronic kidney disease; DM, diabetes mellitus; LV, left ventricle; PAD, peripheral arterial disease.

reduces the patient's ability to tolerate prolonged supine positioning and increases the patient's likelihood of developing further heart failure decompensation with contrast administration and ischemic insults during PCI. This condition can result in both hemodynamic and respiratory decompensation.[20] Arrhythmias, including atrial fibrillation and ventricular tachycardia, as well as underlying valvular lesions affect the patient's hemodynamic status and can be exacerbated during PCI.[21,22] Of particular note is severe aortic stenosis; patients with ischemia (caused in PCI during balloon inflations, atherectomy, and so forth) develop worsening hypotension because of ventricular stunning in the face of a high fixed afterload.

To most accurately evaluate a patient's current hemodynamic status, right heart catheterization is performed at the beginning of a high-risk PCI to characterize the patient's current filling pressures and hemodynamics. Operators are encouraged to begin all high-risk PCIs with a right heart catheterization to reevaluate the patient's filling pressures and biventricular function because the patient's hemodynamic status may have changed since the last interrogation because of ongoing medication titration. In addition, when evaluating the patient's status at the conclusion of a PCI, it can be useful to have preprocedural hemodynamics for comparison.

Factors Specific to Lesion and Procedural Technique

Lesion complexity and anticipated procedural techniques confer important prognostic information when evaluating the risk and anticipated benefits of a coronary intervention. Lesions defined empirically as high complexity include unprotected left main stenosis, heavy calcified or diffuse disease, true bifurcation lesions (Medina 1/1/1, 1/0/1, and 0/1/1), saphenous vein graft lesions, and CTOs.[23,24] Several risk scores have been validated to quantify the anatomic complexity and significance of a patient's coronary artery disease, including the Duke Jeopardy score and the Synergy Between PCI with Taxus and CABG (SYNTAX) score.[25,26]

The Duke Jeopardy score was first described by Califf and colleagues[25] in an effort to predict survival based on the distribution and degree of coronary artery disease. The Duke Jeopardy score estimates the amount of myocardium at risk by dividing the coronary tree into 6 anatomic segments (left anterior descending, first diagonal branch, first septal, left circumflex, first obtuse marginal, and posterior descending artery). Two points are assigned for each segment that has a stenosis 70% or greater, with the addition of 2 points for each downstream segment from a lesion. For example, a significant proximal LAD lesion would have a Jeopardy score of 6 (2 for LAD, 2 for first septal, 2 for diagonal). Jeopardy scores range from 0 to 12, with a score of 2 conferring a 97% 5-year survival and a score of 12 conferring a 55% 5 year survival.

The SYNTAX score was developed to stratify the anatomic complexity of coronary lesions in patients with 3-vessel or left main coronary artery disease to guide surgical versus percutaneous revascularization strategy in a clinical trial.[26] Unlike the Duke Jeopardy score, the SYNTAX score includes lesion characteristics such as calcification, length, ostial location, and bifurcation involvement. In the SYNTAX trial, patients were divided into tertiles of SYNTAX scores, with a score of 22 or lower considered low complexity, 23 to 32 intermediate, and 33 or greater high complexity. The SYNTAX score was further refined with the SYNTAX II score, which combines both anatomic and clinical factors to aid heart team decision making.

Defining high-risk coronary interventions includes an evaluation of anatomic complexity, as exemplified by the Duke Jeopardy score or SYNTAX score. In addition, planned procedural techniques are an important factor in lesion evaluation.[27] Use of atherectomy and prolonged kissing balloon inflations are more likely to induce significant ischemia and hypotension.[28] Use of the retrograde approach in CTO PCI is also associated with higher hemodynamic stress than antegrade CTO PCI because of ischemia to collaterals perfusing the CTO territory and ischemia in the territory of the donor vessel.[29,30] Any lesion involving the last remaining vessel carries high risk of hemodynamic decompensation when ischemia is induced during angioplasty and in the event of any complication involving the last remaining vessel.

HEMODYNAMIC EFFECTS OF MECHANICAL CIRCULATORY SUPPORT IN HIGH-RISK PERCUTANEOUS CORONARY INTERVENTION

The goal of MCS in high-risk PCI is to reduce myocardial oxygen consumption, improve myocardial blood flow, and maintain systemic perfusion during the procedure.[31] Reduced myocardial oxygen consumption and improved myocardial blood flow increase the threshold at which the ventricle becomes ischemic.[32] This condition reduces the adverse effects of myocardial ischemia, including arrhythmias, increased filling pressures caused by diastolic dysfunction, and ultimately systemic hypotension.

Maintaining systemic perfusion with a stable cardiac output and mean arterial pressure prevents the adverse metabolic effects of tissue hypoperfusion that lead to end-organ dysfunction, morbidity, and mortality.

Myocardial oxygen extraction is an efficient process with 70% to 80% of oxygen extracted by myocardial tissue in resting conditions.[33] Because myocardial oxygen extraction is unable to be significantly augmented, changes in myocardial oxygen delivery are primarily driven by coronary blood flow. Coronary blood flow is determined by the systemic pressure, left ventricular end-diastolic pressure, and wall tension. These factors are controlled by the preload, afterload, heart rate, contractility, and wall stress of the ventricle. Imbalance between oxygen supply, as determined by coronary blood flow, and demand results in myocardial ischemia.[34] In general, therapies that reduce afterload or preload, decrease wall stress, or reduce heart rate decrease the myocardial oxygen demand of the ventricle and improve myocardial blood flow, thus reducing the ischemic burden on the heart. The abilities of MCS devices to reduce myocardial oxygen demand and augment coronary blood flow are variable based on the design of each device.[34]

The current MCS devices used in high-risk PCI include the intra-aortic balloon pump (IABP), left ventricle (LV) to aorta assist devices (Impella 2.5, Impella CP, Impella 5.0), left atrium to aorta assist devices (TandemHeart), and venoarterial extracorporeal membrane oxygenation (VA-ECMO). The variable effect on hemodynamics, myocardial oxygen consumption, and cardiac output augmentation of these MCS devices is summarized in **Table 1**.

CURRENT EVIDENCE
Intra-aortic Balloon Pump
As the first widely used percutaneous MCS device, the IABP has enjoyed high rates of use because of widespread availability and ease of use. The IABP has been studied extensively in acute MI with cardiogenic shock (AMICS). Despite its continued use in patients presenting with AMICS, the pivotal IABP-SHOCK II (Intra-aortic Balloon Support for Myocardial Infarction with Cardiogenic Shock) trial found the IABP to not be superior to medical management for the management of cardiogenic shock in patients presenting with acute coronary syndrome.[35]

Within the realm of elective high-risk PCI, several observational trials suggested reduced rates of major adverse cardiac events with upfront IABP insertion compared with ad hoc

Table 1
Hemodynamic effects of commonly used mechanical circulatory support platforms

	Afterload	LVEDP	MAP	CO	Left Ventricular Unloading	Myocardial Oxygen Demand	Maximal Flow (L/min)
IABP	↓	↓	↑	↑	↑	↓	0.5
Impella CP	Variable	↓	↑	↑	↑	↓	4.0
Tandem Heart	⇔	↓	↑	↑	↑	↓	5.0
VA-ECMO	↑	↑ to ⇔	↑	↑	↓	⇔	7.0

Abbreviations: CO, cardiac output; LVEDP, left ventricular end-diastolic pressure; MAP, mean arterial pressure.

IABP insertion. This hypothesis was tested in the Elective Intra-aortic Balloon Conterpulsation During High-risk Percutaneous Coronary Intervention (BCIS-1) trial.[6] The BCIS-1 trial was the first clinical trial to prospectively study MCS in elective high-risk PCI in a randomized fashion. Ultimately, 300 patients were randomized to IABP insertion before high-risk PCI with balloon pump in place for 4 to 24 hours versus standard PCI. The composite end point of MI, death, stroke, or further revascularization at hospital discharge was not significantly different between the groups. Routine IABP use was associated with fewer procedural complications, including periprocedural hypotension and pulmonary edema. However, The routine IABP group had more minor bleeding and access site complications than standard PCI.

Although not powered to examine all-cause mortality, the BCIS-1 cohort was followed for long-term all-cause mortality.[36] The investigators reported a statistically significant reduction in all-cause mortality in the routine IABP group at a median of 51 months after the index procedure. The overall mortality for the cohort was high (33%), reflecting the high-risk patient population enrolled in the BCIS-1 trial. The hazard ratio for all-cause mortality in patients with routine IABP placement before PCI was 0.66, conferring a 34% reduction in all-cause mortality compared with the unsupported PCI group.

Overall, elective IABP insertion in high-risk PCI has a limited role in modern practice. Upfront IABP may be a reasonable option in patients at particularly high risk of hemodynamic decompensation with poor vascular access prohibiting larger device insertion.

Impella
The Impella was first introduced in Europe in 2004. In 2008, the Impella 2.5 became available

in the United States, receiving US Food and Drug Administration (FDA) approval for partial hemodynamic support in cardiac procedures not requiring cardiopulmonary bypass.[37] Since its approval, the Impella has been used in a variety of clinical settings, including cardiogenic shock, acute MI, postcardiotomy syndrome, and high-risk PCI.[38–40] In the subsequent decade, the device has been iterated, with the Impella CP and the Impella 5.0 offering superior cardiac output augmentation and ventricular unloading. The Impella 2.5, CP, and 5.0 have now received FDA approval for procedural use in high-risk PCI as well as in the setting of acute MI and cardiogenic shock.[41]

The Impella system was hypothesized to be superior to IABP in high-risk PCI because of its greater ability to directly unload the ventricle and provide continuous cardiac output, with the Impella 5.0 providing up to 5 L/min compared with the modest contribution of 0.5 L/min with the IABP. The feasibility of Impella-supported high-risk PCI was first prospectively evaluated in the the PROTECT I trial (A prospective feasibility trial investigating the use of the Impella 2.5 system in patients undergoing high-risk percutaneous coronary intervention).[42] Twenty patients undergoing high-risk PCI, defined as unprotected left main or last remaining conduit PCI with an LVEF less than or equal to 35%, underwent Impella 2.5 insertion before PCI. The primary safety end point of major adverse cardiac events, defined as death, MI, target vessel revascularization, urgent CABG, or stroke at 30 days, occurred in 20% of patients. Two patients had increased periprocedural cardiac enzyme levels meeting the definition of MI, and 2 patients expired during the 30 days following the procedure (1 of renal failure leading to cardiac arrest, 1 of sudden cardiac death). Safety end points were reassuring, with the most common complication being access site hematomas in 8 out of 20 patients (although, notably, hemostasis in this trial was achieved with manual compression on the 13-Fr arterial access sites). From an efficacy perspective, all patients were free from hemodynamic compromise during their procedures, and angiographic success was achieved in all patients.

The USpella registry was a multicenter registry designed to evaluate the safety and clinical outcomes of Impella 2.5 in real-world use.[43] In the USpella registry, high-risk PCI was defined at the discretion of the operator and included patients with reduced LV function, complex coronary anatomy, or a high burden of comorbidities. Among the patients who had prophylactic Impella insertion before high-risk PCI to prevent hemodynamic compromise, the rate of overall major adverse cardiac events was 8% with a 96% 30-day survival. The low overall rate of adverse events was notable in light of the anatomic complexity and high-risk nature of the cohort, with an average SYNTAX score of 37%, 56% of patients being surgical turndowns, 66% of patients with New York Heart Association (NYHA) class III or IV symptoms, and 69% of patients with an ejection fraction less than 35%. Secondary safety outcomes were most notable for access site complications (3.4% with access site bleeding requiring transfusion, 3.4% with vascular complications such as dissection or arteriovenous fistula, and 8.6% with hematomas) despite use of endovascular suture-based closure devices. The findings of the USpella registry were encouraging, with clinical outcomes showing 90% success rates in multivessel revascularization, improvement in LVEF, and improvement in NYHA class at discharge. Overall, these results supported the safety and feasibility of the use of Impella 2.5 in high-risk single-vessel and multivessel PCI.

In light of the safety and feasibility of Impella-supported high-risk PCI in PROTECT I and findings suggesting benefit in the USpella registry, the use of the Impella 2.5 versus IABP was studied in patients undergoing high-risk PCI in the prospective, randomized controlled PROTECT II study (A prospective, randomized clinical trial of hemodynamic support with Impella 2.5 versus Intra-Aortic Balloon Pump in patients undergoing high-risk percutaneous coronary intervention).[7] In PROTECT II, patients were eligible for enrollment if they were undergoing elective PCI for unprotected left main, last remaining conduit, or 3-vessel coronary disease with an LVEF less than or equal to 35%. Following iliofemoral angiography to verify anatomic appropriateness for randomization, patients were randomized to

IABP or Impella 2.5 insertion before PCI. The study was concluded early because of futility with a total of 452 patients enrolled in the trial. The patients included in PROTECT II were a high-risk cohort, with 66% of patients with NYHA class III or IV symptoms, an average LVEF of 24%, an average SYNTAX score of 30, and a mean Society of Thoracic Surgeons (STS) mortality of 6%. Notably, there were significant differences in the procedural characteristics between the groups randomized to Impella versus IABP. In procedures among patients randomized to Impella, more contrast was used, more stents were placed, and atherectomy was used more frequently, with a greater duration of use and number of runs. In total, this suggests more extensive and complete coronary revascularization undertaken in the Impella group than in the IABP group.

PROTECT II did not find significant difference in the rate of major adverse events, defined as a composite of all-cause death, MI, stroke, TIA, revascularization procedure, cardiac or vascular operation, acute renal insufficiency, severe intraprocedural hypotension requiring therapy, cardiopulmonary resuscitation, ventricular tachycardia requiring cardioversion, new aortic insufficiency, or angiographic failure of PCI. In the intention-to-treat analysis, there was a 35.1% major adverse event rate in the Impella 2.5 group versus 40.1% in the IABP group ($P = .277$). At 90 days, a trend toward lower major adverse events in the Impella group was noted, although this did not reach statistical significance ($P = .066$). In the per-protocol population, although the 30-day outcomes did not show a significant difference in major adverse events, the 90-day major adverse event rate was significantly lower in the Impella arm (40% vs 51%; $P = .023$). Patients in the Impella group were significantly less likely to undergo repeat revascularization at 90 days compared with the IABP group. Patients in the study showed significant improvements in LVEF and NYHA class, although this did not differ between the Impella and IABP groups.

Overall, the PROTECT II trial was a negative trial. The investigators were not able to show a difference in the primary outcome of major adverse events at 30 days between the patients randomized to Impella versus IABP. However, these findings must be interpreted in the context of variation in procedural techniques used by operators, with more extensive rotational atherectomy and stenting used in the Impella group, likely because of the patients' hemodynamic stability and perceived ability to tolerate more aggressive techniques. This hypothesis fits with the Impella group having higher rates of periprocedural MI at 30 days and lower rates of repeat revascularization at 90 days. In addition, it is unclear whether the high-risk patients in PROTECT II would have been considered candidates for revascularization in the absence of MCS.

TandemHeart

The TandemHeart is a left ventricular assist device that is inserted percutaneously and diverts blood from the left atrium to the femoral artery at up to 5 L/min. Although the need for left atrial access via trans-septal puncture has limited widespread use of this device, several specific clinical settings make the use of TandemHeart attractive, including patients with significant aortic valve disorder or the presence of a left ventricular thrombus. To date, no randomized data has been collected regarding the use of TandemHeart in high-risk PCI.

A prospectively collected single-center registry is the largest published experience describing the use of TandemHeart in high-risk PCI.[44] In this registry from the Mayo clinic, 64 patients underwent high-risk PCI (LVEF<30% and a Duke Jeopardy score of 8 or greater) with TandemHeart over a 5-year period. All of the patients were deemed inoperable because of comorbidities, severity of cardiovascular disease, or both. They were also thought to have a burden of disease and underlying cardiac dysfunction to such a degree than an Impella was considered inadequate periprocedural hemodynamic support. This opinion is reflected in the baseline characteristics of the patient cohort, with an average LVEF of 20%, median SYNTAX score of 33, and median Jeopardy score of 10. Many of these patients had a recent MI (52%) complicated by periprocedural cardiogenic shock (29%), with 45% of patients already having an IABP in place before intervention.

Despite the high coronary complexity and high risk of this group, there was a 97% procedural success rate, with left main intervention in 62% of patients and rotational atherectomy in 48% of patients. The 30-day survival in this high-risk group was 90%. The most common adverse event was vascular complications (13% of patients), which largely occurred in the early experience. The rates of access site complications decreased markedly with the routine assessment of iliofemoral access as a component of case selection and procedure planning.

A meta-analysis by Briasoulis and colleagues[45] included 8 cohort studies with a total of 205 patients that received TandemHeart for high-risk PCI. Short-term mortality was 8%, with major bleeding rates of 3.6%. These outcomes are in line with prior studies given the high-risk nature of the group being studied.

Overall, the limited data available supports the use of TandemHeart for MCS in select high-risk PCI. The high rates of 30-day mortality and vascular complications may at least in part be explained by the selection bias among these observational studies; patients with Tandem-Heart placement were considered to need more hemodynamic support than could be provided by an Impella and were likely sicker at baseline. Despite this, observational data have shown acceptable safety and feasibility in TandemHeart placement for high-risk PCI in this inoperable cohort of patients.

Venoarterial Extracorporeal Membrane Oxygenation

Data for elective high-risk PCI on ECMO are limited to small single-center experiences. Brilakis and colleagues[46] describe their experience with 5 patients over the course of 5 years who underwent high-risk PCI with ECMO support. The patients underwent PCI for LV systolic dysfunction (4 patients) or non-ST elevation MI (1 patient). All interventions were technically successful. The most common adverse event was vascular access complications, with 1 pseudoaneurysm requiring surgical repair and 2 femoral hematomas. All of their patients lived through 1-year follow-up with a mean increase in LVEF of 24%.

Similar findings were reported by Barbarash and colleagues,[47] whose experience with elective high-risk PCI with ECMO support included 12 inoperable patients in 1 year. In this group, all PCI procedures were technically successful and no in-hospital major adverse events were observed. There were minimal vascular complications in this case series, with only 1 femoral hematoma reported. Six-month follow-up was notable for 100% survival, with 2 patients requiring repeat revascularization.

These single-center reports suggest that ECMO-supported PCI is feasible and can be performed safely in a highly selected group of patients in experienced centers.

CLINICAL DECISION MAKING

Clinical decision making for patients undergoing high-risk PCI requires a nuanced understanding of the complex interplay between patient,

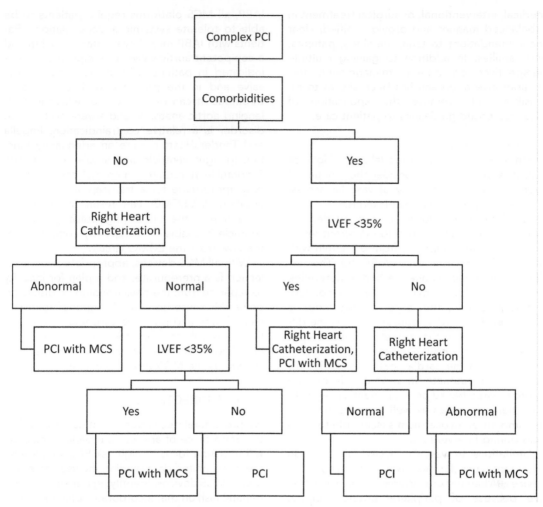

Fig. 5. Algorithm for decision making in the use of MCS for patients undergoing elective high-risk PCI. Patients entering the algorithm are those undergoing complex PCI, defined as procedures with high potential for ischemia, including Duke Jeopardy score greater than 8, last remaining conduit, multivessel obstructive disease, left main bifurcation with planned atherectomy, retrograde CTO, and those in which an unanticipated complication such as no reflow or dissection would likely result in hemodynamic collapse. Comorbidities include significant valvular lesions, prior diagnosis of heart failure, chronic kidney disease, advanced age, and frailty.

lesion, and hemodynamic characteristics as well as the unique assets and liabilities of the available MCS modalities. Although general conclusions can be drawn from the available randomized and observational data, these must be weighed carefully against patient-specific and procedure-specific considerations. Although several decision-making algorithms have been proposed (Fig. 5), none have been prospectively validated.

Heart Team Approach
The heart team, a multidisciplinary group convened to discuss complex patient care

decisions, was initially established in clinical trials as a way to select appropriate patients for interventional versus surgical revascularization. The heart team is composed at a minimum of the patient's primary cardiologist, consulting interventional cardiologist, and consulting cardiac surgeon. Similar to the manner in which the heart team has become the standard of care in aortic valve disease, a heart team for coronary artery disease has been proposed as the standard of care for patients being evaluated for high-risk revascularization.[12] These teams use a comprehensive patient assessment to weigh the relative risks and benefits of medical, interventional, or surgical treatment in a balanced manner and provide unified, clear recommendations to team members, patients, and families. In addition to gaining multiple perspectives on patient management, this collaborative approach has been shown to be feasible and promote the application of evidence-based guidelines to patient care.[48]

Device Selection

When selecting an MCS modality for high-risk PCI, it is important to consider the amount of support needed, adequacy of vascular access, and device-specific contraindications.

As detailed previously in this article, the available MCS devices provide different levels of hemodynamic support, from 0.5 L/min with IABP to 5 to 6 L/min with VA-ECMO. The cardiac output deficit is one method to determine the amount of hemodynamic support needed. In this paradigm, the target cardiac index is 2.2 L/min. The cardiac output deficit is the difference between the target cardiac output and the cardiac output nadir during the procedure. Although the cardiac output nadir is only possible to estimate in advance, it can be approximated based on the patient's preprocedure hemodynamics as well as an estimate of the amount of myocardium susceptible to stunning during intervention.

Limitations in vascular access are also an important consideration when choosing MCS devices. When femoral arterial access is prohibitive because of peripheral arterial disease, excessive tortuosity, or small patient habitus, alternative access (subclavian cutdown or percutaneous axillary access) has been shown to be feasible and safe for both IABP and Impella CP.[49–51] Severe peripheral arterial disease can be prohibitive when considering larger sheaths for blood return for TandemHeart or VA-ECMO. A novel approach in patients requiring large-bore access for ECMO, TandemHeart, or Impella 5.0 with inadequate transfemoral access is transcaval access, which allows venous transfemoral access with the sheath traversing the inferior vena cava to the abdominal aorta by means of percutaneous access.[52,53] Although this novel approach has allowed a class of patients who previously would have been ineligible for MCS to undergo these procedures, its use is limited by the small number of operators with adequate skills for percutaneous transcaval access, management, and removal.

In addition, device-specific contraindications must be considered when choosing an appropriate MCS platform. With the exception of the IABP, all MCS platforms require patients to be able to tolerate systemic anticoagulation.[5] Patients with IABP must have a stable rhythm and a competent aortic valve. The Impella is contraindicated in patients with a mechanical aortic valve and in the presence of left ventricular thrombus. It can be difficult to deliver in challenging aortic anatomy, and severe aortic valve disorder is a relative contraindication. Impella and TandemHeart require an adequately functioning right ventricle and stable rhythm. The TandemHeart requires interatrial septum anatomy appropriate for a transseptal puncture. In addition, VA-ECMO can result in ventricular distention if the underlying pulsatility of the ventricle is unable to adequately compete with the flow from the ECMO circuit.[5]

With all MCS devices, appropriate patient selection is a prerequisite, and a plan for inability to separate from the device should be discussed before MCS insertion with the input of advanced heart failure and palliative care team members. It is critical to monitor for complications including limb ischemia, stroke, and bleeding as long as the MCS device is in place.

FUTURE DIRECTIONS

As procedural techniques continue to evolve, the importance of appropriate patient selection will remain a focus in high-risk PCI. At present, there are limited data guiding the use and selection of MCS devices. Identifying patients in a systematic fashion that incorporates patient, lesion, and hemodynamic factors is critical to advancing clinical research. Clinically, more sophisticated methods for patient selection will allow identification of the patients who are the most likely to benefit from intervention as well as those in whom high-risk PCI is futile.

SUMMARY

Overall, the growing technical complexity of modern PCI combined with the increasingly comorbid elderly population has resulted in an expanding group of patients who are considered inoperable or high risk for CABG. These patients, identified based on their comorbidities, lesion characteristics, and hemodynamic state, represent a cohort who now are offered high-risk PCI with the use of MCS. To date, clinical research has not conclusively shown benefit to the routine use of MCS in prospective randomized controlled trials. Ongoing research focusing on identifying the appropriate patient/lesion to derive the greatest benefit with MCS-facilitated high-risk PCI is critical to the growth of this field. In addition, lower-profile, more powerful devices that maximize hemodynamic benefits while minimizing vascular complications will be critical to making MCS more efficacious in this group of patients and interventions.

CLINICS CARE POINTS

- Identifying patients who are high risk for hemodynamic collapse during elective high-risk PCI requires understanding of patient-specific risk factors, hemodynamics, and lesion/procedural technique factors. Patients with multiple comorbidities and decompensated hemodynamics who require advanced interventional techniques, including kissing balloons, atherectomy, or use of last remaining conduit, should be strongly considered for MCS.

- The most widely used device in the United States for high-risk PCI is the IABP. The IABP has a low risk of vascular complications, but provides minimal augmentation in forward systemic flow.

- The LV to aortic assist device (Impella) has grown in use given the ease of use, effectiveness of ventricular unloading, and stable increases in cardiac output with this device. Vascular complications remain an important complication limiting the clinical benefit of these devices.

- The use of TandemHeart and VA-ECMO to support high-risk PCI has been shown to be safe and feasible in limited observational data.

- Future directions for research in high-risk PCI will likely focus on identifying the group of patients most likely to benefit from MCS-supported PCI.

DISCLOSURES

The authors have no relevant disclosures to report.

REFERENCES

1. Nowbar AN, Gitto M, Howard JP, et al. Mortality from ischemic heart disease. Circ Cardiovasc Qual Outcomes 2019;12(6):e005375.
2. Mensah GA, Wei GS, Sorlie PD, et al. Decline in cardiovascular mortality: possible causes and implications. Circ Res 2017;120(2):366–80.
3. Bass TA. High-risk percutaneous coronary interventions in modern day clinical practice: current concepts and challenges. Circ Cardiovasc Interv 2015; 8(12):e003405.
4. Atkinson TM, Ohman EM, O'Neill WW, et al. A practical approach to mechanical circulatory support in patients undergoing percutaneous coronary intervention: an interventional perspective. JACC Cardiovasc Interv 2016;9(9):871–83.
5. Rihal CS, Naidu SS, Givertz MM, et al. 2015 SCAI/ACC/HFSA/STS clinical expert consensus statement on the use of percutaneous mechanical circulatory support devices in cardiovascular care: endorsed by the American Heart Association, the Cardiological Society of India, and Sociedad Latino Americana de Cardiologia Intervencion; Affirmation of Value by the Canadian Association of Interventional Cardiology-Association Canadienne de Cardiologie d'intervention. J Am Coll Cardiol 2015;65(19):e7–26.
6. Perera D, Stables R, Thomas M, et al. Elective intra-aortic balloon counterpulsation during high-risk percutaneous coronary intervention: a randomized controlled trial. JAMA 2010;304(8):867–74.
7. O'Neill WW, Kleiman NS, Moses J, et al. A prospective, randomized clinical trial of hemodynamic support with Impella 2.5 versus intra-aortic balloon pump in patients undergoing high-risk percutaneous coronary intervention: the PROTECT II study. Circulation 2012;126(14):1717–27.
8. Escaned J, Collet C, Ryan N, et al. Clinical outcomes of state-of-the-art percutaneous coronary revascularization in patients with de novo three vessel disease: 1-year results of the SYNTAX II. Eur Heart J 2017;38(42):3124–34.
9. Nashef SA, Roques F, Sharples LD, et al. EuroSCORE II. Eur J Cardiothorac Surg 2012;41(4):734–45.
10. Waldo SW, Secemsky EA, O'Brien C, et al. Surgical ineligibility and mortality among patients with unprotected left main or multivessel coronary artery disease undergoing percutaneous coronary intervention. Circulation 2014;130(25):2295–301.
11. McNulty EJ, Ng W, Spertus JA, et al. Surgical candidacy and selection biases in nonemergent left main stenting: implications for observational studies. JACC Cardiovasc Interv 2011;4(9):1020–7.
12. Riley RF, Henry TD, Mahmud E, et al. SCAI position statement on optimal percutaneous coronary interventional therapy for complex coronary artery disease. Catheter Cardiovasc Interv 2020;96:346–62.
13. Hwang JK, Lee SH, Song YB, et al. Glycemic control status after percutaneous coronary intervention and long-term clinical outcomes in patients with type 2 diabetes mellitus. Circ Cardiovasc Interv 2017;10(4):e004157.
14. Enriquez JR, de Lemos JA, Parikh SV, et al. Association of chronic lung disease with treatments and

outcomes patients with acute myocardial infarction. Am Heart J 2013;165(1):43–9.

15. Sarnak MJ, Amann K, Bangalore S, et al. Chronic kidney disease and coronary artery disease: JACC state-of-the-art review. J Am Coll Cardiol 2019; 74(14):1823–38.

16. Wallace TW, Berger JS, Wang A, et al. Impact of left ventricular dysfunction on hospital mortality among patients undergoing elective percutaneous coronary intervention. Am J Cardiol 2009;103(3):355–60.

17. Parikh SV, Saya S, Divanji P, et al. Risk of death and myocardial infarction in patients with peripheral arterial disease undergoing percutaneous coronary intervention (from the National Heart, Lung and Blood Institute Dynamic Registry). Am J Cardiol 2011;107(7):959–64.

18. Klein LW, Block P, Brindis RG, et al. Percutaneous coronary interventions in octogenarians in the American College of Cardiology-National Cardiovascular Data Registry: development of a nomogram predictive of in-hospital mortality. J Am Coll Cardiol 2002;40(3):394–402.

19. Brennan JM, Curtis JP, Dai D, et al. Enhanced mortality risk prediction with a focus on high-risk percutaneous coronary intervention: results from 1,208,137 procedures in the NCDR (National Cardiovascular Data Registry). JACC Cardiovasc Interv 2013;6(8):790–9.

20. Steg PG, Kerner A, Van de Werf F, et al. Impact of in-hospital revascularization on survival in patients with non-ST-elevation acute coronary syndrome and congestive heart failure. Circulation 2008;118:1163–71.

21. Sutton NR, Seth M, Ruwende C, et al. Outcomes of patients with atrial fibrillation undergoing percutaneous coronary intervention. J Am Coll Cardiol 2016;68(9):895–904.

22. Mehta RH, Starr AZ, Lopes RD, et al. Incidence of and outcomes associated with ventricular tachycardia or fibrillation in patients undergoing primary percutaneous coronary intervention. JAMA 2009; 301(17):1779–89.

23. Ilis SG, Guetta V, Miller D, et al. Relation between lesion characteristics and risk with percutaneous intervention in the stent and glycoprotein IIb/IIIa era: an analysis of results from 10,907 lesions and proposal for new classification scheme. Circulation 1999; 100(19):1971–6.

24. Krone RJ, Shaw RE, Klein LW, et al. Evaluation of the American College of Cardiology/American Heart Association and the Society for Coronary Angiography and Interventions lesion classification system in the current "stent era" of coronary interventions (from the ACC-National Cardiovascular Data Registry). Am J Cardiol 2003;92(4):389–94.

25. Califf RM, Phillips HR 3rd, Hindman MC, et al. Prognostic value of a coronary artery jeopardy score. J Am Coll Cardiol 1985;5(5):1055–63.

26. Serruys PW, Morice MC, Kappetein AP, et al. Percutaneous coronary intervention versus coronary-artery bypass grafting for severe coronary artery disease. N Engl J Med 2009;360(10):961–72 [published correction appears in N Engl J Med 2013; 368(6):584].

27. Patel MR, Calhoon JH, Dehmer GJ, et al. ACC/AATS/AHA/ASE/ASNC/SCAI/SCCT/STS 2016 appropriate use criteria for coronary revascularization in patients with acute coronary syndromes: a report of the American College of Cardiology Appropriate Use Criteria Task Force, American Association for Thoracic Surgery, American Heart Association, American Society of Echocardiography, American Society of Nuclear Cardiology, Society for Cardiovascular Angiography and Interventions, Society of Cardiovascular Computed Tomography, and the Society of Thoracic Surgeons. J Nucl Cardiol 2017;24(2):439–63.

28. Meraj PM, Shlofmitz E, Kaplan B, et al. Clinical outcomes of atherectomy prior to percutaneous coronary intervention: a comparison of outcomes following rotational versus orbital atherectomy (COAP-PCI study). J Interv Cardiol 2018;31(4): 478–85.

29. Chen SL, Santoso T, Zhang JJ, et al. Clinical outcome of double kissing crush versus provisional stenting of coronary artery bifurcation lesions: the 5-year follow-up results from a randomized and multicenter DKCRUSH-II Study (Randomized Study on Double Kissing Crush Technique Versus Provisional Stenting Technique for Coronary Artery Bifurcation Lesions). Circ Cardiovasc Interv 2017; 10(2):e004497.

30. Sapontis J, Salisbury AC, Yeh RW, et al. Early procedural and health status outcomes after chronic total occlusion angioplasty: a report from the OPEN-CTO Registry (Outcomes, Patient Health Status, and Efficiency in Chronic Total Occlusion Hybrid Procedures). JACC Cardiovasc Interv 2017; 10(15):1523–34.

31. Naidu SS. Novel percutaneous cardiac assist devices: the science of and indications for hemodynamic support. Circulation 2011;123(5):533–43.

32. Chatterjee K. Coronary hemodynamics in heart failure and effects of therapeutic interventions. J Card Fail 2009;15(2):116–23.

33. Goodwill AG, Dick GM, Kiel AM, et al. Regulation of coronary blood flow. Compr Physiol 2017;7(2): 321–82.

34. Burkhoff D, Naidu SS. The science behind percutaneous hemodynamic support: a review and comparison of support strategies. Catheter Cardiovasc Interv 2012;80(5):816–29.

35. Thiele H, Zeymer U, Neumann FJ, et al. Intraaortic balloon pump support for myocardial infarction with cardiogenic shock. N Engl J Med 2012;367:1287–96.

36. Perera D, Stables R, Clayton T, et al. Long-term mortality from the balloon pump-assisted coronary intervention study (BCIS-1). Circulation 2013;127:207–12.

37. Basir MB, Kapur NK, Patel K, et al. Improved outcomes associated with the use of shock protocols: updates from the national cardiogenic shock initiative. Catheter Cardiovasc Interv 2019;93:1173–83.

38. Henriques JP, Remmelink M, Baan J, et al. Safety and feasibility of elective high-risk percutaneous coronary intervention procedures with left ventricular support of the Impella Recover LP 2.5. Am J Cardiol 2006;97:990–2.

39. Siegenthaler MP, Brehm K, Strecker T, et al. The Impella Recover microaxial left ventricular assist device reduces mortality for postcardiotomy failure: a three-center experience. J Thorac Cardiovasc Surg 2004;127(3):812–22.

40. O'Neill WW, Schreiber T, Wohns DH, et al. The current use of Impella 2.5 in acute myocardial infarction complicated by cardiogenic shock: results from the USpella Registry. J Interv Cardiol 2014;27(1):1–11.

41. Aggarwal B, Aman W, Jeroudi O, et al. Mechanical circulatory support in high-risk percutaneous coronary intervention. Methodist Debakey Cardiovasc J 2018;14(1):23–31.

42. Dixon SR, Henriques JPS, Mauri L, et al. A prospective feasibility trial investigating the use of the Impella 2.5 system in patients undergoing high-risk percutaneous coronary intervention. JACC Cardiovasc Interv 2009;2:91–6.

43. Maini B, Naidu SS, Mulukutla S, et al. Real-world use of the Impella 2.5 circulatory support system in complex high-risk percutaneous coronary intervention: the USpella Registry. Catheter Cardiovasc Interv 2012;80:717–25.

44. Alli OO, Singh IM, Holmes DR, et al. Percutaneous left ventricular assist device with TandemHeart for high-risk percutaneous coronary intervention: The Mayo Clinic Experience. Catheter Cardiovasc Interv 2012;80:728–34.

45. Briasoulis A, Telila T, Palla M, et al. Meta-analysis of usefulness of percutaneous left ventricular assist devices for high-risk percutaneous coronary interventions. Am J Cardiol 2016;118:369–75.

46. Shaukat A, Hryniewicz-Czeneszew K, Sun B, et al. Outcomes of extracorporeal membrane oxygenation support for complex high-risk elective percutaneous coronary interventions: a single-center experience and review of the literature. J Invasive Cardiol 2018;30(12):456–60.

47. Tomasello SD, Boukhris M, Ganyukov V, et al. Outcome of extracorporeal membrane oxygenation support for complex high-risk elective percutaneous coronary interventions: a single center experience. Heart Lung 2015;44:309–13.

48. Young MN, Kolte D, Cadigan ME, et al. Multidisciplinary heart team approach for complex coronary artery disease: Single center clinical presentation. J Am Heart Assoc 2020;9(8):e014738.

49. Estep JD, Cordero-Reyes AM, Bhimaraj A, et al. Percutaneous placement of an intra-aortic balloon pump in the left axillary/subclavian position provides safe, ambulatory long-term support as bridge to heart transplantation. JACC Heart Fail 2013;1(5):382–8.

50. Mathur M, Hira RS, Smith BM, et al. Fully percutaneous technique for transaxillary implantation of the impella CP. JACC Cardiovasc Interv 2016;9(11):1196–8.

51. Dawson K, Jones TL, Kearney KE, et al. Emerging role of large-bore percutaneous axillary vascular access: a step-by-step guide. Interv Cardiol 2020;15:e07.

52. Gaudard P, Mourad M, Eliet J, et al. Management and outcome of patients supported with Impella 5.0 for refractory cardiogenic shock. Crit Care 2015;19:363.

53. Frisoli TM, Guerrero M, O'Neill WW. Mechanical circulatory support with Impella to facilitate percutaneous coronary intervention for post-TAVI bilateral coronary obstruction. Catheter Cardiovasc Interv 2016;88(1):e34–7.

Mechanical Circulatory Support in Cardiogenic Shock due to Structural Heart Disease

Pedro Villablanca, MD, MSc*, Paul Nona, MD,
Alejandro Lemor, MD, MSc, Mohammed Qintar, MD, MSc,
Brian O'Neill, MD, James Lee, MD, Tiberio Frisoli, MD,
Dee Dee Wang, MD, Marvin H. Eng, MD,
William W. O'Neill, MD

KEYWORDS

- Cardiogenic shock • Mechanical circulatory support • Aortic stenosis • Aortic regurgitation
- Mitral regurgitation • Mitral stenosis

KEY POINTS

- Early recognition and escalation of care with mechanical circulatory support are crucial for patients presenting with cardiogenic shock due to structural heart disease.
- Selection of mechanical circulatory support methods should be based on device availability, familiarity of the multidisciplinary team with the device, and specific needs of the patient.
- Surgical or transcatheter repair of structural heart disease should be done using appropriate mechanical support with a "heart team" approach after the patient has improved.

Tremendous advances in all forms of cardiovascular care[1] have developed over the past decade, with remarkable and dramatic declines in cardiovascular mortality (between 60% and 70%).[2] Despite such advances in cardiovascular disease therapies, cardiogenic shock (CS) is a common cause of mortality, and management of CS remains challenging. Acute coronary syndrome accounts for more than 80% of cases of CS.[3] As a result, interest in CS has predominantly focused on managing acute coronary syndrome, including revascularization. Few studies to date have explored the role of structural heart disease (SHD) in the pathogenesis of CS. In the SHOCK (should we emergently revascularize occluded coronaries for cardiogenic shock) trial registry of 1190 patients with CS, 8% of patients

had SHD that caused or worsened their hemodynamic status, with a mortality close to 100%.[4] Similar poor outcomes have been observed in other observational studies.[5–7]

Temporary mechanical circulatory support (MCS) is an attractive and intuitive option to use when other medical therapies have been insufficient. Many exciting developments in MCS methods have occurred in the past few years, including the development of smaller portable pumps.[8] Although the field is a growing one, patients with SHD are often excluded from randomized trials, and the role of mechanical therapies in this specific population remains controversial and not well established.

Department of Structural Heart Disease, Division of Cardiology, Henry Ford Health System, 2799 West Grand Boulevard, CFP 4th Floor, Detroit, MI 48202, USA
* Corresponding author. Center for Structural Heart Disease, Henry Ford Hospital, 2799 West Grand Boulevard, CFP 4th Floor, Detroit, MI 48202.
E-mail address: PVillab1@hfhs.org

Intervent Cardiol Clin 10 (2021) 221–234
https://doi.org/10.1016/j.iccl.2020.12.007
2211-7458/21/

SHD refers to non–coronary heart disease for which some therapy, surgical or percutaneous, exists. Examples include valvular heart disease, congenital disorders, mechanical complication of acute myocardial infarction, and cardiomyopathies.[9] Although the treatment of SHD often requires pharmacologic and surgical intervention, established and emerging device-based interventions in the setting of CS offer exceptional promise for revolutionizing the practice of cardiovascular medicine. Nevertheless, when patients with SHD present with CS, treatment becomes more challenging and complex.

Currently, there are no published guidelines for using MCS in patients with SHD. The focus of this review is on MCS device selection, specifically, selection pathways for patients with CS from SHD. The objective is to provide the reader with an understanding of general considerations, based on current evidence and institutional experience, for determining the appropriateness of MCS for SHD.

HEART TEAM

With the number of therapeutic options increasing, the "heart team" has become an increasingly important strategy for evaluating SHD, whereby comprehensive decision making may result in a change of diagnostic or therapeutic strategies and promote improved outcomes. Several guidelines have highlighted the effect of heart teams for managing valvular heart disease and heart failure.[10–14] Determining an optimal treatment strategy for patients with complex SHD and CS requires assessing each patient's presenting illness, clinical stability, anatomy, comorbidities, and goals of care. Implementing the scarce guidance available to guide SHD-CS management to the nuances of real-world practice can be challenging; thus, supporting an interdisciplinary model of care is key.

DEFINITION OF CARDIOGENIC SHOCK

The American Heart Association defines CS as a state in which ineffective cardiac output caused by a primary cardiac disorder results in both clinical and biochemical manifestations of inadequate tissue perfusion and dysfunction. In addition to severe systolic and diastolic cardiac dysfunction compromising macrocirculation and microcirculation, systemic inflammatory response syndrome and even sepsis may develop, which could result in multiorgan dysfunction syndrome and biochemical manifestations of inadequate tissue perfusion, such

as elevated arterial lactate. The most common hemodynamic criteria for CS include a systolic blood pressure less than 90 mm Hg, a cardiac index less than 2.2 L/min/m,[2] a pulmonary capillary wedge pressure greater than 18 mm Hg, or a right ventricular (RV) end diastolic pressure greater than 10 to 15 mm Hg. Although myocardial infarction with left ventricular (LV) failure remains the most common cause of CS, any acute cause of severe LV or RV dysfunction may lead to CS.[15]

HEMODYNAMIC MONITORING

Although not mandatory in clinical practice, assessing objective hemodynamic parameters, such as reduced cardiac index and elevated pulmonary capillary wedge pressure, is helpful for diagnosing CS, and other hemodynamic parameters are essential for defining RV function in CS.[16] A large national US registry showed that assessing premature atrial contractions in patients with CS is an effective strategy, and using this method is associated with improved outcomes, which may reflect better selection of patients or better use of the information to guide therapies.[17] To improve patient outcomes, the authors recommend assessing hemodynamic parameters using premature atrial contractions in patients with SHD-CS for monitoring guiding treatment effectiveness.

MEDICAL THERAPY

Disease management in patients with CS should focus on maintaining adequate cardiac output for vital end-organ perfusion. For patients with acute coronary syndrome with CS, therapy for patient-specific cause should focus on coronary reperfusion and treatment of the underlying SHD that is causing the CS or is a consequence of myocardial infarction. Urgent revascularization and surgical/transcatheter therapies remain the gold standard of care for CS; however, patients often are unstable with increased mortality to receive a definitive therapy. SHD-specific definitive interventions will not be discussed because they are beyond the scope of this review.

Pharmacotherapies, such as inotropes and vasopressors, are used to enhance contractility and modulate vascular tone. Maximal medical therapy (volume resuscitation, vasodilators, inotropic agents) is not considered a justifiable endpoint for refractory CS, at least in well-resourced health settings.[18] The lack of clear evidence on the effectiveness of pharmacologic inotropic support and the limited (or adverse) effect of catecholamine therapy on survival in patients with CS from acute myocardial infarction[19,20] are the driving forces behind exploration of mechanical means of circulatory support.[21]

The authors believe that physicians treating patients with SHD should adhere to recommendations similar to those recently proposed by the European Acute Cardiovascular Care Association for patients with acute coronary syndrome complicated by CS, such as the following: (1) When severe SHD is diagnosed and is contributing to instability, the patient should be admitted or transferred to a hospital that has 24/7 MCS capability to treat the impending cardiovascular crisis; (2) catecholamine and inotropes should be administered at the lowest possible dose and for the shortest possible duration; (3) the routine use of intra-aortic balloon pump is not recommended, whereas the use of percutaneous MCS devices should be restricted to cases of refractory CS, with treatment being guided by individual physician experience in dedicated centers; and (4) in addition to the general principles of RV dysfunction management, the use of MCS devices with dedicated RV support or venous arterial extracorporeal membrane oxygenation (VA-ECMO) may be considered for certain patients with refractory CS.[22]

MECHANICAL CIRCULATORY SUPPORT OPTIONS

Temporary selection of MCS should be based on device availability, familiarity of the multidisciplinary team with the device, and specific patient needs.[8] In the United States, temporary percutaneous mechanical options for drug-refractory CS have included the following methods: intra-aortic balloon pump, counterpulsation, and percutaneous LV assist devices. Specific LV assist devices include the Tandem-Heart percutaneous system (Cardiac Assist, Inc, Pittsburgh, PA, USA), the Impella (Abiomed Europe GmbH, Aachen, Germany), and VA-ECMO.[23] A variant of VA-ECMO is left atrial venoarterial extracorporeal membrane oxygenation (LAVA-ECMO), which is a novel technique that involves transseptal placement of a single multistage drainage venous femoral cannula to simultaneously drain both atria in patients with severe LV systolic dysfunction.[24] For RV failure, right-sided support devices, such as Impella RP and the TandemHeart RA-PA, are available options in addition to ECMO.[23] **Fig. 1** shows schematic drawings of current percutaneous mechanical support devices for CS, including technical features.

AORTIC STENOSIS

Aortic stenosis is the most common valvular heart disease causing LV outflow tract obstruction. Pressure gradient and LV pressure overload are the hallmarks of severe aortic stenosis that cause leaflet stretch, fluid shear stress, bending stresses, and pressure forces. This tissue damage results in elevated left atrial pressure and pulmonary capillary wedge pressure. Over time, some patients may develop LV dysfunction because of increased wall stress secondary to inadequate wall thickening, potentially resulting in "afterload mismatch."[25,26] Patients with severe aortic stenosis, LV dysfunction, and unrevascularized coronary artery disease are particularly susceptible to hemodynamic decompensation owing to limited myocardial reserve.[27]

The incidence of CS in patients with aortic stenosis is low (close to 6%),[28] but mortality in patients who have developed CS can be considerably high, up to 70%, if no durable intervention is performed.[29] Therapeutic interventions for CS related to aortic stenosis are challenging because of a paucity of data. Whereas medical treatment alone is an unreliable option, and surgery is often deemed prohibitive, it is unclear whether direct transcatheter aortic valve replacement (TAVR) or balloon aortic valvuloplasty (BAV) followed by elective TAVR or surgical aortic valve replacement (SAVR) after medical stabilization should be performed. Medical therapy for patients with aortic stenosis and CS should include optimal ventilatory and inotropic support, and every effort should be made to identify and treat the precipitating factors. Treatment options for aortic stenosis with CS include surgery or urgent TAVR.[30] Despite recent advances in therapies, caring for patients with severe aortic stenosis who go on to develop systolic dysfunction and CS remains an important clinical challenge, and this condition is associated with increased morbidity and mortality.[30,31]

Over the past decade, Impella has become commercially available for providing circulatory support in patients with aortic stenosis.[32] A relative contraindication for using the Impella device is a concern about potential compromise of blood flow in the remaining valvular orifice from the presence of a catheter, which could lead to worsened hemodynamics through a severely stenotic aortic valve orifice. Regardless,

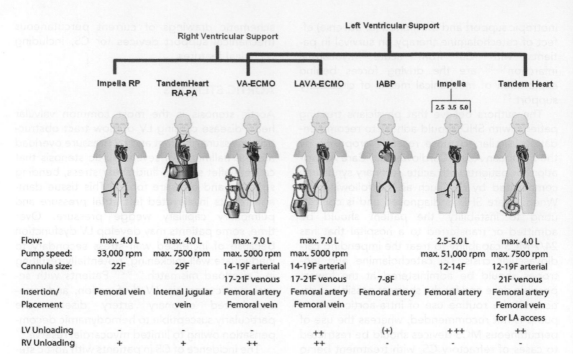

	Right Ventricular Support			**Left Ventricular Support**			
	Impella RP	TandemHeart RA-PA	VA-ECMO	LAVA-ECMO	IABP	Impella	Tandem Heart
						2.5 3.5 5.0	
Flow:	max. 4.0 L	max. 4.0 L	max. 7.0 L	max. 7.0 L		2.5-5.0 L	max. 4.0 L
Pump speed:	33,000 rpm	max. 7500 rpm	max. 5000 rpm	max. 5000 rpm		max. 51,000 rpm	max. 7500 rpm
Cannula size:	22F	29F	14-19F arterial	14-19F arterial		12-14F	12-19F arterial
			17-21F venous	17-21F venous	7-8F		21F venous
Insertion/	Femoral vein	Internal jugular	Femoral artery	Femoral artery	Femoral artery	Femoral artery	Femoral artery
Placement		vein	Femoral vein	Femoral vein			Femoral vein
							for LA access
LV Unloading	-	-	-	++	(+)	+++	++
RV Unloading	+	+	++	++	-	-	-

Fig. 1. Current percutaneous mechanical support devices for CS. IABP, intra-aortic balloon pump. (*Adapted from* Thiele H, Ohman EM, de Waha-Thiele S, Zeymer U, Desch S. Management of cardiogenic shock complicating myocardial infarction: an update 2019. *Eur Heart J.* 2019;40(32):2671-2683; with permission.)

the use of Impella has been shown to be feasible, with promising results seen in selected patients with severe aortic stenosis.[33] The Impella device directly aspirates blood from the LV into the aorta in series with the native cardiac blood flow. Owing to the unique design, this device effectively unloads the LV and simultaneously stabilizes the patient's hemodynamics and augments cardiac output. Implantation of the 2.5, 3.5, and 5.0 left-sided Impella seems to be feasible in patients with severe aortic stenosis, and a balloon-assist technique may be used to facilitate device implantation when initial unassisted attempts have failed. Improved hemodynamic stability may enhance the tolerability of lengthy and complex procedures by unloading the LV.[34,35] In cases of CS with concomitant coronary artery disease, the risk of the decompensation is higher,[36] but MCS with Impella can improve distal coronary pressure and coronary perfusion pressures in the presence of critical coronary stenosis.[37] **Fig. 2A** shows schematic drawings of current percutaneous mechanical support devices for aortic stenosis in CS.

Several single-center studies have demonstrated the feasibility of using BAV as a bridge to TAVR and SAVR in patients with acute presentations and as a way to triage select high-risk

patients who are not good candidates for aortic valve replacement.[38,39] When BAV is performed and the ventricles are paced at high rates, a sudden decrease in stroke volume and cardiac output causing ischemic and hemodynamic strain may result during the procedure, and these results may be due to periods of hypotension with subsequent systemic and coronary hypoperfusion. BAV can be done with the Impella device in place to minimize interruption of blood flow during balloon inflation and during high-risk BAV[40,41] (**Fig. 3**). Furthermore, evidence exists that points to a similar cerebrovascular risk in patients undergoing BAV or TAVR, with the central venous access device registry reporting an adverse event rate of 1.72% at 30 days following Impella-assisted BAV.[36]

Peri-interventional CS is associated with high mortality and can occur during TAVR in a variety of scenarios, such as coronary obstruction, refractory ventricular arrhythmia, annular rupture, and hemodynamic collapse.[33,42] In a study of 54 patients who required an MCS device during TAVR, Impella was used in only 7 patients: 3 elective cases and 4 emergency rescues. The overall in-hospital mortality in this study was 11% for elective cases and 53% for emergency rescue. CS was the cause of death in 50% of cases, and all-cause mortality at 1 year was

A Aortic Stenosis

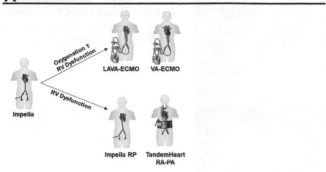

B Aortic Regurgitation

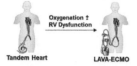

C Mitral Stenosis

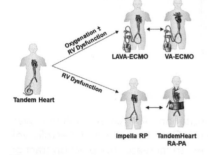

D Mitral Regurgitation

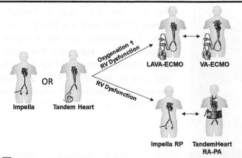

E Ventricular Septal Defect

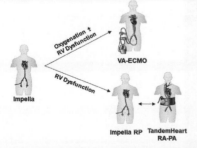

Fig. 2. Recommended algorithm for MCS utilization for SHD: (*A*) aortic stenosis, (*B*) AR, (*C*) mitral stenosis, (*D*) mitral regurgitation, and (*E*) VSD.

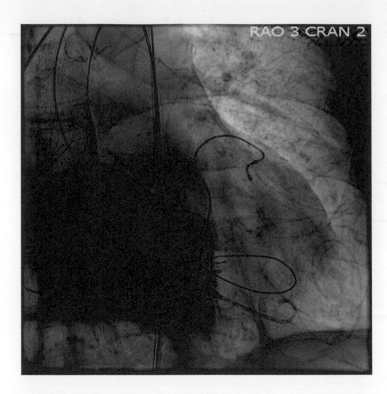

Fig. 3. Impella CP device-assisted BAV in a patient with CS and severe aortic stenosis. (*Courtesy of* ABIOMED Inc., Danvers, MA.)

19% for elective cases and 71% for emergency cases.[43] In situations wherein Impella has not been available, ECMO has been used for bailout in TAVR use complicated by CS[44] (**Fig. 4**).

AORTIC REGURGITATION

Aortic regurgitation (AR) causes volume overload of the LV. Over time, LV end-diastolic volume continues to increase; the ejection fraction

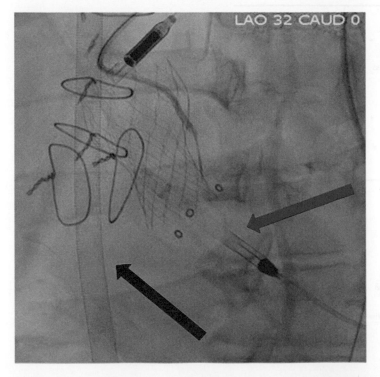

Fig. 4. Combined use of percutaneous ECMO and Impella CP in a case of periprocedural coronary occlusion in a valve-in-valve TAVI (*blue arrow*: venous ECMO cannula; *red arrow*: Impella CP in the left ventricle). (Impella CP courtesy of ABIOMED Inc., Danvers, MA.)

drops, and these changes may precede the appearance of clinical symptoms. Acute AR can be life threatening, as LV dilatation and other compensatory mechanisms cannot develop rapidly enough to prevent hemodynamic deterioration. Regarding the medical management of AR in the setting of CS, stabilization with airway intubation and hemodynamic support may be required, especially before intervention. The use of vasodilators, such as nitroprusside, in conjunction with inotropic therapy may help with hemodynamic stabilization.[45] Pacing after BAV and TAVR has been adopted as temporary or permanent therapy to mitigate perivalvular leak in patients affected by moderate to severe AR.[46] This approach is based on the concept that a shorter diastolic phase reduces the time available for blood to flow back into the ventricle, thus diminishing the ventricular overload. Prompt SAVR remains the standard of care for operable patients; however, TAVR has been used in selective cases.[47]

Unfortunately, given the pathophysiology of the disease, most (if not all) MCS have a relative contraindication in the setting of severe AR. Management of CS with acute AR with an Impella or intra-aortic balloon pump device would not provide adequate circulatory support or mitigate aortic insufficiency. If MCS is

mandated, the TandemHeart device could be considered, although it indirectly unloads LV volume by actively unloading the left atrium; however, the AR may remain unaffected or could be worsened because of pressurized blood in the aorta, increasing the retrograde flow. At the authors' center, they have used Tandem-Heart as a bridge to surgery, considering the limitations mentioned above. Case reports describing use of TandemHeart with off-label use of an Amplatzer occluder device to limit AR have reported mitigation of the acute phase as a bridge to surgery.[48] Another possibility for treating severe AR is the LAVA-ECMO, as it might be better for unloading the LV than the standard VA-ECMO because it offers sufficient biventricular decompression.

MITRAL STENOSIS

The incidence of CS in patients with mitral stenosis is unknown but is probably very low in wealthier nations, despite being a highly prevalent condition worldwide. It occurs mainly in patients who have not received treatment until the mitral stenosis is very advanced, with CS being the final manifestation. Mortality can reach close to 25% if it is not treated accordingly. The key hemodynamic consequence of mitral stenosis is the development of a

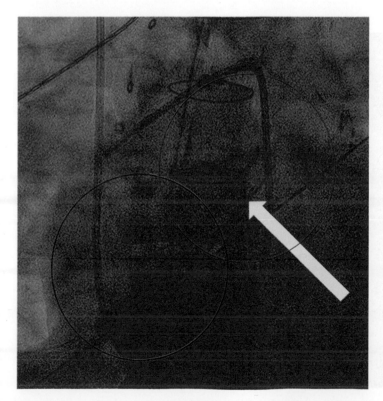

Fig. 5. LAVA ECMO in a patient with biventricular failure and severe mitral regurgitation. The multistage cannula (*arrow*) drains in both the left atrium via end hole (*red circle*) and right atrium via side holes (*blue circle*).

pressure gradient between the left atrium and LV, which is transmitted to the pulmonary circulation and results in an increase in both pulmonary pressures and pulmonary vascular resistance, resulting in pulmonary edema, RV failure, and CS. A rapid diagnosis of this condition is important because emergency interventions, such as valve replacement or percutaneous balloon mitral valvuloplasty (PBMV), are effective and readily available. Only a few case series have reported successful treatment of CS with PBMV.[49–51] The most commonly encountered occurrence is an underlying mitral stenosis affected by septic or hypovolemic shock, which may trigger CS.

Medical treatments to stabilize patients with mitral stenosis include optimal ventilatory and inotropic support. Excessive tachycardia in these patients shortens diastole and causes an undesired increase in pressure gradients across the mitral valve. When a patient's condition remains unstable despite treatment of precipitating factors, emergent mechanical relief of mitral stenosis should be done as soon as possible with either PBMV or surgery. If inappropriate valvular anatomy precludes PBMV or surgery, or if a contraindication for PMBV exists, the device of choice should be TandemHeart. This MCS facilitates hemodynamic stabilization by directly unloading the left atrium and promoting decongestion of the lungs, which facilitates a bridge to

mitral valve surgery. If there is RV failure and hypoxemia, the CS mitral stenosis can be treated with VA-ECMO, with the preferred use of the LAVA-ECMO modality that decompresses both atriums and pulmonary filling pressures.

MITRAL REGURGITATION

Acute mitral regurgitation is a rare but lethal condition that often results in CS and high mortality, especially in the setting of acute coronary syndrome (10% to 40% with surgery; 80% without surgery).[4,52,53] Urgent surgical mitral repair or replacement is the current standard of care; however, a significant portion of patients do not receive surgery because of prohibitive operative risk or inability to be stabilized before surgery.[4,54] As a result, large randomized studies of this phenomenon are difficult to perform, and evidence of treatment is limited to case reports, even for the current gold standard of surgery.[53,55] MitraClip has been previously reported for treating acute mitral regurgitation after myocardial infarction or with CS, with most cases being poor LV function.[56–60]

Recently improved MCS could potentially stabilize patients with acute mitral regurgitation and serve as a bridge to definitive treatment.[61] The preoperative implantation of MCS seems to improve outcomes in patients with CS who are

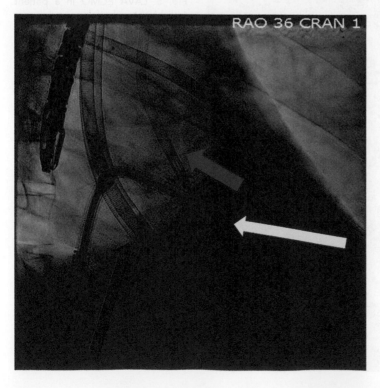

RAO 36 CRAN 1

Fig. 6. Combined use of percutaneous TH-RAPA and Impella CP in a case of severe mitral regurgitation secondary to chordae rupture post myocardial infarction treated percutaneously with edge-to-edge repair (*blue arrow*: venous TH-RAPA cannula; *red arrow*: Impella CP in the left ventricle; *yellow arrow*: MitraClip system). (TandemHeart RAPA courtesy of TandemLife; LivaNova, London, UK; Impella CP courtesy of ABIOMED Inc., Danvers, MA; MitraClip courtesy of Abbott Vascular, Santa Clara, CA, USA).

suitable for urgent surgery[62,63] and is generally accepted as the standard of care until emergent mitral valve surgery can be performed. The intra-aortic balloon pump has been a commonly used device, although it offers the least cardiac output augmentation; however, it is widely available and can decrease afterload, thereby supporting adequate mean arterial pressure and potentially decreasing the mitral regurgitation. The Impella device, used alone or together with ECMO (ie, ECPELLA), offers more significant cardiac output augmentation and directly unloads the LV. On the other hand, ECMO has been less commonly used alone, as it may increase total peripheral vascular resistance, potentially worsening the mitral regurgitation. In cases whereby only ECMO is available, physicians should consider the LAVA-ECMO modality to unload the left atrium (Fig. 5). The TandemHeart device can directly unload the left atrium and potentially offer the best hemodynamic effect in patients with acute mitral regurgitation. However, MCS use has not been without risk, and it has been reported to directly cause chordal rupture and acute mitral regurgitation after myocardial infarction.[64]

POSTMYOCARDIAL INFARCTION VENTRICULAR SEPTAL DEFECT

Ventricular septal defect or rupture (VSD) is an infrequent but lethal complication of acute myocardial infarction.[65] When VSD is associated with CS, the mortality is greater than 80%.[66] The definitive therapy for VSD is surgical repair or use of percutaneous closure devices for eligible patients.[67] Inotropes and vasopressors worsen left-to-right shunting, whereas vasodilators decrease shunting at the expense of worsening hypotension. Frequently, very ill patients with VSD and CS will need hemodynamic stabilization with MCS to improve systemic perfusion. Most of the available MCS devices, including intra-aortic balloon pump,[68] ECMO,[69,70] Tandem-Heart,[71,72] and Impella (including 5.0 support), have been used to treat unstable patients with VSD and CS.[73,74] Despite widespread use of percutaneous MCS, guidelines for optimal use have not been defined because the low incidence and high acuity of VSD have made randomized clinical studies almost impossible to conduct. The European Society of Cardiology Guidelines categorize VSD with CS as a class IIa recommendation (level of evidence C) and suggest using short-term MCS therapy as a bridge to recovery or surgery; however, the guidelines do not specify a preferred form of support.[75]

A computer-simulation model assessing hemodynamic effects of MCS in VSD showed that no form of MCS could normalize hemodynamics in the setting of VSD whereby blood flow through the pulmonary artery (PA) was always markedly elevated. This hemodynamic

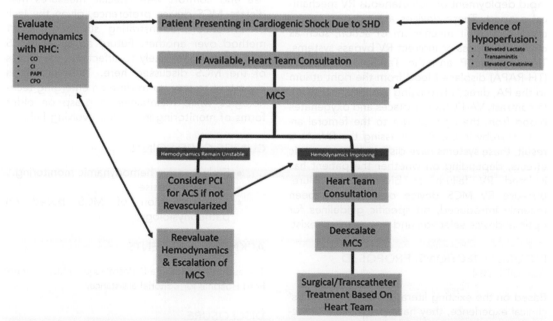

Fig. 7. Proposed algorithm for hemodynamic monitoring and initiation of MCS in those patients presenting with CS due to SHD. ACS, acute coronary syndrome; CI, cardiac index; CO, cardiac output; CPO, cardiac power output; PAPI, pulmonary artery pulsatility index; PCI, primary cutaneous intervention; RHC, right heart catherization.

phenomenon may occur because of increased left-to-right shunting through the VSD or increased right-sided venous return from increased systemic flow in the presence of left-sided support provided by the MCS device. However, this model showed that a combination of 2 devices can provide the greatest degree of overall circulatory support while simultaneously unloading the LV (ie, ECPELLA), with the Impella 5.0 being the most effective MCS and the intra-aortic balloon pump being the least effective MCS.[76] One clinical feature that favors use of an ECMO approach is significant hypoxemia.

RIGHT-SIDED STRUCTURAL HEART DISEASE

CS secondary to isolated right-sided SHD is rare, as this disease can be well tolerated over time. However, left-sided SHD commonly manifests with right RV failure, which increases short-term mortality.[77,78] Diagnosing acute RV failure remains a major clinical challenge. Physical examination, echocardiography, and laboratory tests are helpful tools; however, assessment of premature atrial contractions with other well-established indexes of RV failure can help to confirm diagnosis. Intra-aortic balloon pumps are commonly used to treat RV failure but are not optimally suited for this purpose. Recent advances in percutaneous technology have brought multiple devices into practice that allow rapid deployment of percutaneous RV mechanical support. These devices are categorized according to their mechanism of action, such as direct RV bypass or indirect RV bypass systems. The Impella RP and the TandemHeart RAPA (TH-RAPA) displace blood from the right atrium to the PA, directly bypassing the RV[79,80] (Fig. 6). In contrast, VA-ECMO displaces and oxygenates blood from the right atrium to the femoral artery, thereby indirectly bypassing the RV. As a result, these systems have distinct hemodynamic effects, depending on whether the patient has isolated RV failure or biventricular failure. Because RV MCS device options have been recently introduced, no specific guidelines for optimal device selection and management exist.

FUTURE DIRECTIONS: PROPOSED ALGORITHM

Based on the existing literature and the authors' clinical experience, they have proposed and recommended an algorithm for the use of MCS devices for each SHD discussed in this review (Fig. 2). To guide the management of CS owing to SHD, the authors encourage adopting an early consultation with the heart team to determine an optimal management strategy on a case-by-case basis. They advocate the recognition of CS and early use of percutaneous MCS when indicated based on objective hemodynamic and perfusion parameters to prevent progressive deterioration and organ hypoperfusion. Defining which MCS is the best option should be determined by the main underlying condition and the presence or absence of RV failure and/or hypoxemia. MCS may be considered a temporizing therapy for transcatheter options or potentially as a bridge to surgery or transplant after patient stabilization (Fig. 7).

SUMMARY

Treatment of SHD in the setting of CS remains challenging. Many advances have improved diagnosis and therapy for SHD in CS. Early use of MCS devices instead of dose escalation of inotropes and vasopressors might prevent disease progression and reduce mortality in patients with SHD complicated with CS. Appropriate device selection is still a complex decision-making process, and the authors expect that ongoing studies that take into account the severity of CS, goals of care, patient-specific risks, technical limitations, and assessment for futility of care will help develop better recommendations for MCS choice. Local expertise and comfort with specific measures may dictate MCS device preference, given the lack of evidence demonstrating superiority of 1 method over another. Future advances in CS management are likely to affect the usefulness of the MCS discussed here. Therefore, it is important to stay up-to-date on emerging technologies while maintaining a grasp on older forms of monitoring in an ever-evolving field.

CLINICS CARE POINTS

- Early invasive hemodynamic monitoring.
- Center expertise.
- Early adoption of MCS based on pathophysiology.

ACKNOWLEDGMENTS

The authors thank Karla D Passalacqua, PhD, at Henry Ford Hospital for editorial assistance.

DISCLOSURE

Dr Eng is a clinical proctor for Edwards Lifesciences, Medtronic and Boston Scientific. Dr Frisoli is a clinical proctor for Edwards Lifesciences, Abbott, Boston Scientific, and Medtronic. Dr B O'Neill has served as a consultant and received research support from Edwards Lifesciences. Dr Lee is a consultant for Heart-Flow. Dr W. O'Neill has served as a consultant for Abiomed, Edwards Lifesciences, Medtronic, Boston Scientific, Abbott Vascular and St. Jude Medical; and serves on the Board of Directors of Neovasc Inc. Dr Wang is a consultant to Edwards Lifesciences, Boston Scientific, receives research grant support from Boston Scientific assigned to employer Henry Ford Health System, is a member of the Edwards CLASP IITR, Steering Committee, and Abbott PARADIGM Steering Committee. All other authors report no relevant financial disclosures.

REFERENCES

1. Nabel EG, Braunwald E. A tale of coronary artery disease and myocardial infarction. N Engl J Med 2012;366(1):54–63.

2. Mensah GA, Wei GS, Sorlie PD, et al. Decline in cardiovascular mortality: possible causes and implications. Circ Res 2017;120(2):366–80.

3. Harjola VP, Lassus J, Sionis A, et al. Clinical picture and risk prediction of short-term mortality in cardiogenic shock. Eur J Heart Fail 2015;17(5):501–9.

4. Thompson CR, Buller CE, Sleeper LA, et al. Cardiogenic shock due to acute severe mitral regurgitation complicating acute myocardial infarction: a report from the SHOCK Trial Registry. SHould we use emergently revascularize Occluded Coronaries in cardiogenic shocK? J Am Coll Cardiol 2000;36(3 Suppl A):1104–9.

5. Fox AC, Glassman E, Isom OW. Surgically remediable complications of myocardial infarction. Prog Cardiovasc Dis 1979;21(6):461–84.

6. Yamanishi H, Izumoto H, Kitahara H, et al. Clinical experiences of surgical repair for mitral regurgitation secondary to papillary muscle rupture complicating acute myocardial infarction. Ann Thorac Cardiovasc Surg 1998;4(2):83–6.

7. Cercek B, Shah PK. Complicated acute myocardial infarction. Heart failure, shock, mechanical complications. Cardiol Clin 1991;9(4):569–93.

8. Peura JL, Colvin-Adams M, Francis GS, et al. Recommendations for the use of mechanical circulatory support: device strategies and patient selection: a scientific statement from the American Heart Association. Circulation 2012;126(22):2648–67.

9. DeMaria AN. Structural heart disease? J Am Coll Cardiol 2014;63(6):603–4.

10. Vahanian A, Alfieri O, Andreotti F, et al. Guidelines on the management of valvular heart disease (version 2012): the Joint Task Force on the Management of Valvular Heart Disease of the European Society of Cardiology (ESC) and the European Association for Cardio-Thoracic Surgery (EACTS). Eur J Cardiothorac Surg 2012;42(4):S1–44.

11. Ponikowski P, Voors AA, Anker SD, et al. 2016 ESC Guidelines for the diagnosis and treatment of acute and chronic heart failure: the Task Force for the diagnosis and treatment of acute and chronic heart failure of the European Society of Cardiology (ESC). Developed with the special contribution of the Heart Failure Association (HFA) of the ESC. Eur J Heart Fail 2016;18(8):891–975.

12. Authors/Task Force members, Windecker S, Kolh P, et al. 2014 ESC/EACTS Guidelines on myocardial revascularization: the Task Force on Myocardial Revascularization of the European Society of Cardiology (ESC) and the European Association for Cardio-Thoracic Surgery (EACTS) developed with the special contribution of the European Association of Percutaneous Cardiovascular Interventions (EAPCI). Eur Heart J 2014;35(37):2541–619.

13. Kabrhel C, Jaff MR, Channick RN, et al. A multidisciplinary pulmonary embolism response team. Chest 2013;144(5):1738–9.

14. Kolte D, Parikh SA, Piazza G, et al. Vascular teams in peripheral vascular disease. J Am Coll Cardiol 2019;73(19):2477–86.

15. van Diepen S, Katz JN, Albert NM, et al. Contemporary management of cardiogenic shock: a scientific statement from the American Heart Association. Circulation 2017;136(16):e232–68.

16. Kapur NK, Esposito ML, Bader Y, et al. Mechanical circulatory support devices for acute right ventricular failure. Circulation 2017;136(3):314–26.

17. Hernandez GA, Lemor A, Blumer V, et al. Trends in utilization and outcomes of pulmonary artery catheterization in heart failure with and without cardiogenic shock. J Card Fail 2019;25(5):364–71.

18. Shekar K, Gregory SD, Fraser JF. Mechanical circulatory support in the new era: an overview. Crit Care 2016;20:66.

19. Dunser MW, Hasibeder WR. Sympathetic overstimulation during critical illness: adverse effects of adrenergic stress. J Intensive Care Med 2009; 24(5):293–316.

20. Overgaard CB, Dzavik V. Inotropes and vasopressors: review of physiology and clinical use in cardiovascular disease. Circulation 2008;118(10):1047–56.

21. Reynolds HR, Hochman JS. Cardiogenic shock: current concepts and improving outcomes. Circulation 2008;117(5):686–97.

22. Zeymer U, Bueno H, Granger CB, et al. Acute Cardiovascular Care Association position statement for the diagnosis and treatment of patients with acute myocardial infarction complicated by cardiogenic shock: a document of the Acute Cardiovascular Care Association of the European Society of Cardiology. Eur Heart J Acute Cardiovasc Care 2020;9(2): 183–97.

23. Thiele H, Ohman EM, de Waha-Thiele S, et al. Management of cardiogenic shock complicating myocardial infarction: an update 2019. Eur Heart J 2019;40(32):2671–83.

24. Choi MS, Sung K, Cho YH. Clinical pearls of venoarterial extracorporeal membrane oxygenation for cardiogenic shock. Korean Circ J 2019;49(8):657–77.

25. Ross J Jr. Afterload mismatch and preload reserve: a conceptual framework for the analysis of ventricular function. Prog Cardiovasc Dis 1976;18(4):255–64.

26. Gunther S, Grossman W. Determinants of ventricular function in pressure-overload hypertrophy in man. Circulation 1979;59(4):679–88.

27. Paradis JM, Fried J, Nazif T, et al. Aortic stenosis and coronary artery disease: what do we know? What don't we know? A comprehensive review of the literature with proposed treatment algorithms. Eur Heart J 2014;35(31):2069–82.

28. Percutaneous balloon aortic valvuloplasty. Acute and 30-day follow-up results in 674 patients from the NHLBI Balloon Valvuloplasty Registry. Circulation 1991;84(6):2383–97.

29. Buchwald AB, Meyer T, Scholz K, et al. Efficacy of balloon valvuloplasty in patients with critical aortic stenosis and cardiogenic shock–the role of shock duration. Clin Cardiol 2001;24(3):214–8.

30. Kolte D, Khera S, Vemulapalli S, et al. Outcomes following urgent/emergent transcatheter aortic valve replacement: insights from the STS/ACC TVT Registry. JACC Cardiovasc Interv 2018;11(12):1175–85.

31. Elbadawi A, Elgendy IY, Mentias A, et al. Outcomes of urgent versus nonurgent transcatheter aortic valve replacement. Catheter Cardiovasc Interv 2020;96(1):189–95.

32. Martinez CA, Singh V, Londono JC, et al. Percutaneous retrograde left ventricular assist support for interventions in patients with aortic stenosis and left ventricular dysfunction. Catheter Cardiovasc Interv 2012;80(7):1201–9.

33. Singh V, Mendirichaga R, Inglessis-Azuaje I, et al. The role of Impella for hemodynamic support in patients with aortic stenosis. Curr Treat Options Cardiovasc Med 2018;20(6):44.

34. Spiro J, Venugopal V, Raja Y, et al. Feasibility and efficacy of the 2.5 L and 3.8 L Impella percutaneous left ventricular support device during high-risk, percutaneous coronary intervention in patients with severe aortic stenosis. Catheter Cardiovasc Interv 2015;85(6):981–9.

35. Johnson DW, Erwin IJ. Use of Impella 5.0 prior to transcatheter aortic valve replacement in a patient with severe aortic stenosis and cardiogenic shock. J Heart Valve Dis 2017;26(4):485–7.

36. Singh V, Yadav PK, Eng MH, et al. Outcomes of hemodynamic support with Impella in very high-risk patients undergoing balloon aortic valvuloplasty: results from the Global cVAD Registry. Int J Cardiol 2017;240:120–5.

37. Alqarqaz M, Basir M, Alaswad K, et al. Effects of Impella on coronary perfusion in patients with critical coronary artery stenosis. Circ Cardiovasc Interv 2018;11(4):e005870.

38. Ben-Dor I, Maluenda G, Dvir D, et al. Balloon aortic valvuloplasty for severe aortic stenosis as a bridge to transcatheter/surgical aortic valve replacement. Catheter Cardiovasc Interv 2013;82(4):632–7.

39. Saia F, Marrozzini C, Moretti C, et al. The role of percutaneous balloon aortic valvuloplasty as a bridge for transcatheter aortic valve implantation. EuroIntervention 2011;7(6):723–9.

40. Megaly M, Jones P. Impella CP-assisted balloon aortic valvuloplasty. J Cardiol Cases 2016;14(2):49–51.

41. Ludeman DJ, Schwartz BG, Burstein S. Impella-assisted balloon aortic valvuloplasty. J Invasive Cardiol 2012;24(1):E19–20.

42. Almalla M, Kersten A, Altiok E, et al. Hemodynamic support with Impella ventricular assist device in patients undergoing TAVI: a single center experience. Catheter Cardiovasc Interv 2020;95(3):357–62.

43. Singh V, Damluji AA, Mendirichaga R, et al. Elective or emergency use of mechanical circulatory support devices during transcatheter aortic valve replacement. J Interv Cardiol 2016;29(5):513–22.

44. Uehara K, Minakata K, Saito N, et al. Use of extracorporeal membrane oxygenation in complicated transcatheter aortic valve replacement. Gen Thorac Cardiovasc Surg 2017;65(6):329–36.

45. Nishimura RA, Otto CM, Bonow RO, et al. 2014 AHA/ACC guideline for the management of patients with valvular heart disease: executive summary: a report of the American College of Cardiology/American Heart Association Task Force on Practice Guidelines. J Am Coll Cardiol 2014;63(22):2438–88.

46. Ali O, Salinger MH, Levisay JP, et al. High pacing rates for management of aortic insufficiency after balloon aortic valvuloplasty or transcatheter aortic valve replacement. Catheter Cardiovasc Interv 2014;83(1):162–8.

47. Yoon SH, Schmidt T, Bleiziffer S, et al. Transcatheter aortic valve replacement in pure native aortic valve regurgitation. J Am Coll Cardiol 2017;70(22):2752–63.

48. Pollak P, Lim DS, Kern J. Management of severe aortic regurgitation in a patient with cardiogenic shock using a percutaneous left ventricular assist device and transcatheter occlusion of the failed aortic valve homograft as a bridge to surgical valve replacement. Catheter Cardiovasc Interv 2014;83(1):E141–5.

49. Lokhandwala YY, Banker D, Vora AM, et al. Emergent balloon mitral valvotomy in patients presenting with cardiac arrest, cardiogenic shock or refractory pulmonary edema. J Am Coll Cardiol 1998;32(1):154–8.

50. Patel JJ, Munclinger MJ, Mitha AS, et al. Percutaneous balloon dilatation of the mitral valve in critically ill young patients with intractable heart failure. Br Heart J 1995;73(6):555–8.

51. Goldman JH, Slade A, Clague J. Cardiogenic shock secondary to mitral stenosis treated by balloon mitral valvuloplasty. Cathet Cardiovasc Diagn 1998;43(2):195–7.

52. Russo A, Suri RM, Grigioni F, et al. Clinical outcome after surgical correction of mitral regurgitation due to papillary muscle rupture. Circulation 2008; 118(15):1528–34.

53. Schroeter T, Lehmann S, Misfeld M, et al. Clinical outcome after mitral valve surgery due to ischemic papillary muscle rupture. Ann Thorac Surg 2013; 95(3):820–4.

54. O'Gara PT, Kushner FG, Ascheim DD, et al. 2013 ACCF/AHA guideline for the management of ST-elevation myocardial infarction: a report of the American College of Cardiology Foundation/ American Heart Association Task Force on Practice Guidelines. J Am Coll Cardiol 2013;61(4): e78–140.

55. Bouma W, Wijdh-den Hamer IJ, Koene BM, et al. Predictors of in-hospital mortality after mitral valve surgery for post-myocardial infarction papillary muscle rupture. J Cardiothorac Surg 2014;9:171.

56. Chan V, Messika-Zeitoun D, Labinaz M, et al. Percutaneous mitral repair as salvage therapy in patients with mitral regurgitation and refractory cardiogenic shock. Circ Cardiovasc Interv 2019;12(11):e008435.

57. Cheng R, Dawkins S, Hamilton MA, et al. Percutaneous mitral repair for patients in cardiogenic shock requiring inotropes and temporary mechanical circulatory support. JACC Cardiovasc Interv 2019;12(23):2440–1.

58. Estevez-Loureiro R, Settergren M, Winter R, et al. Effect of gender on results of percutaneous edge-to-edge mitral valve repair with MitraClip system. Am J Cardiol 2015;116(2):275–9.

59. Hernández-Enríquez M, Freixa X, Sanchis L, et al. MitraClip® repair in cardiogenic shock due to acute mitral regurgitation: from near-death to walking. J Heart Valve Dis 2018;27(1):114–6.

60. Seizer P, Schibilsky D, Sauter R, et al. Percutaneous mitral valve edge-to-edge repair assisted by hemodynamic support devices: a case series of bailout procedures. Circ Heart Fail 2017;10(5):e004051.

61. Rab T, Ratanapo S, Kern KB, et al. Cardiac shock care centers: JACC review topic of the week. J Am Coll Cardiol 2018;72(16):1972–80.

62. DiVita M, Visveswaran GK, Makam K, et al. Emergent TandemHeart-ECMO for acute severe mitral regurgitation with cardiogenic shock and hypoxaemia: a case series. Eur Heart J Case Rep 2020;4(1): 1–6.

63. Jalil B, El-Kersh K, Frizzell J, et al. Impella percutaneous left ventricular assist device for severe acute ischaemic mitral regurgitation as a bridge to surgery. BMJ Case Rep 2017;2017. bcr2017219749.

64. Bhatia N, Richardson TD, Coffin ST, et al. Acute mitral regurgitation after removal of an Impella device. Am J Cardiol 2017;119(8):1290–1.

65. Singh V, Rodriguez AP, Bhatt P, et al. Ventricular septal defect complicating ST-elevation myocardial infarctions: a call for action. Am J Med 2017;130(7): 863.e1-2.

66. Lemery R, Smith HC, Giuliani ER, et al. Prognosis in rupture of the ventricular septum after acute myocardial infarction and role of early surgical intervention. Am J Cardiol 1992;70(2):147–51.

67. Murday A. Optimal management of acute ventricular septal rupture. Heart 2003;89(12):1462–6.

68. Thiele H, Lauer B, Hambrecht R, et al. Short- and long-term hemodynamic effects of intra-aortic balloon support in ventricular septal defect complicating acute myocardial infarction. Am J Cardiol 2003;92(4):450–4.

69. Rob D, Spunda R, Lindner J, et al. A rationale for early extracorporeal membrane oxygenation in patients with postinfarction ventricular septal rupture complicated by cardiogenic shock. Eur J Heart Fail 2017;19(Suppl 2):97–103.

70. Kwon J, Lee D. The effectiveness of extracorporeal membrane oxygenation in a patient with post myocardial infarct ventricular septal defect. J Cardiothorac Surg 2016;11(1):143.

71. Gregoric ID, Bieniarz MC, Arora H, et al. Percutaneous ventricular assist device support in a patient with a postinfarction ventricular septal defect. Tex Heart Inst J 2008;35(1):46–9.

72. Gregoric ID, Mesar T, Kar B, et al. Percutaneous ventricular assist device and extracorporeal membrane oxygenation support in a patient with postinfarction ventricular septal defect and free wall rupture. Heart Surg Forum 2013;16(3):E150–1.

73. Ibebuogu UN, Bolorunduro O, Hwang I. Impella-assisted transcatheter closure of an acute postinfarction ventricular septal defect. BMJ Case Rep 2016;2016. bcr2015213887.

74. La Torre MW, Centofanti P, Attisani M, et al. Posterior ventricular septal defect in presence of cardiogenic shock: early implantation of the Impella recover LP 5.0 as a bridge to surgery. Tex Heart Inst J 2011;38(1):42–9.

75. McMurray JJ, Adamopoulos S, Anker SD, et al. ESC guidelines for the diagnosis and treatment of acute and chronic heart failure 2012: the Task Force for

the Diagnosis and Treatment of Acute and Chronic Heart Failure 2012 of the European Society of Cardiology. Developed in collaboration with the Heart Failure Association (HFA) of the ESC. Eur J Heart Fail 2012;14(8):803–69.

76. Pahuja M, Schrage B, Westermann D, et al. Hemodynamic effects of mechanical circulatory support devices in ventricular septal defect. Circ Heart Fail 2019;12(7):e005981.

77. Zehender M, Kasper W, Kauder E, et al. Right ventricular infarction as an independent predictor of prognosis after acute inferior myocardial infarction. N Engl J Med 1993;328(14):981–8.

78. Jacobs AK, Leopold JA, Bates E, et al. Cardiogenic shock caused by right ventricular infarction: a report from the SHOCK registry. J Am Coll Cardiol 2003;41(8):1273–9.

79. Anderson MB, Goldstein J, Milano C, et al. Benefits of a novel percutaneous ventricular assist device for right heart failure: the prospective RECOVER RIGHT study of the Impella RP device. J Heart Lung Transplant 2015;34(12):1549–60.

80. Ravichandran AK, Baran DA, Stelling K, et al. Outcomes with the tandem Protek duo dual-lumen percutaneous right ventricular assist device. ASAIO J 2018;64(4):570–2.

Temporary Mechanical Circulatory Support as a Bridge to Heart Transplant or Durable Left Ventricular Assist Device

Sonali Arora, MD[a], Auras R. Atreya, MD[b],
Edo Y. Birati, MD[c,d,e], Supriya Shore, MD, MSCS[f,g,*]

KEYWORDS

- Cardiogenic shock • End-stage heart failure • Impella • TandemHeart • ECMO • CentriMag
- Rotaflow • ProtekDuo • IABP

KEY POINTS

- Temporary mechanical circulatory support is being increasingly used as a bridge to advanced therapies for patients with heart failure.
- A wide array of devices is available for both right and left ventricle support. Each device has its own hemodynamic blueprint.
- The timely identification of cardiogenic shock and the use of shock teams are potential strategies that can improve survival in patients with heart failure and cardiogenic shock.
- The choice of device should be based on patient needs and the comfort level of the clinical team managing the patient.

INTRODUCTION

Heart failure (HF) is a chronic, progressive condition with a prevalence of more than 6 million in the United States.[1,2] The current understanding is that 5% of hospitalized patients have end-stage HF,[3] and it is associated with a high financial burden on the health care system and a mortality rate of 75% at 1 year.[4] Accordingly, for patients with stage D HF, consideration of advanced HF therapies such as durable a left ventricular assist device (LVAD) or heart transplantation (HT) is

indicated. These patients may require temporary mechanical circulatory support (TMCS) as a bridge to advanced HF therapies. Cardiogenic shock presents as a spectrum and can be classified into stages A to E depending on severity (Fig. 1).

PERCUTANEOUS TEMPORARY MECHANICAL CIRCULATORY SUPPORT FOR THE LEFT VENTRICLE

Currently available forms of percutaneous TMCS for cardiogenic shock in stage D HF supporting

[a] Institute of Heart and Lung Transplant, Krishna Institute of Medical Sciences Hospitals, 1-8-31/1, Minister Road, Krishna Nagar Colony, Secunderabad, Telangana 500003, India; [b] Interventional Cardiology, AIG Institute of Cardiac Sciences and Research, 1, Mindspace Road, Gachibowli, Hyderabad, Telangana 500032, India; [c] Division of Cardiovascular Medicine, University of Pennsylvania, Philadelphia, PA 19104, USA; [d] Division of Cardiovascular Medicine, Poriya Medical Center, Israel 152801; [e] Perelman Center for Advanced Medicine, 11th Floor, South Tower, 3400 Civic Center Boulevard, Philadelphia, PA 19104, USA; [f] Department of Internal Medicine, Division of Cardiovascular Disease, University of Michigan, Ann Arbor, MI 48103, USA; [g] University of Michigan, North Campus Research Complex, 2800 Plymouth Road, 16-169C, Ann Arbor, MI 48109, USA
* Corresponding author. University of Michigan, North Campus Research Complex, 2800 Plymouth Road, 16-169C, Ann Arbor, MI 48109.
E-mail address: shores@umich.edu

Intervent Cardiol Clin 10 (2021) 235–249
https://doi.org/10.1016/j.iccl.2020.12.011
2211-7458/21/© 2021 Elsevier Inc. All rights reserved.

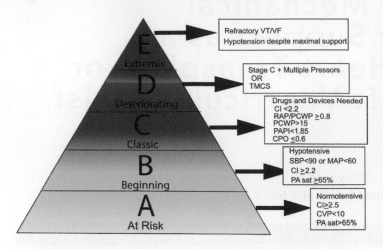

Fig. 1. Stages of cardiogenic shock based on the Society for Cardiovascular Angiography and Interventions (SCAI) classification. CI, cardiac index; CPO, cardiac power output; MAP, mean arterial pressure; PA, pulmonary artery; PAPI, pulmonary artery pressure index; PCWP, pulmonary capillary wedge pressure; RAP, right atrial pressure; SBP, systolic blood pressure; TMCS, temporary mechanical circulatory support; VF, ventricular fibrillation; VT, ventricular tachycardia. (Baran DA, Grines CL, Bailey S, et al. SCAI clinical expert consensus statement on the classification of cardiogenic shock: This document was endorsed by the American College of Cardiology (ACC), the American Heart Association (AHA), the Society of Critical Care Medicine (SCCM), and the Society of Thoracic Surgeons (STS) in April 2019. Catheter Cardiovasc Interv 2019;94(1):29-37. doi: 10.1002/ccd.28329. Epub 2019 May 19. PMID: 31104355; with permission.)

the left ventricle (LV) can be broadly classified based on the hemodynamic circuit as (i) LV to aorta assist devices, namely, the intra-aortic balloon pump and the Impella; (ii) left atrium (LA) to systemic artery, namely, the Tandem Heart; and (iii) the right atrium (RA) to systemic artery, namely, venoarterial extracorporeal membrane oxygenation (VA-ECMO; **Fig. 2**). To date, there are no large-scale randomized trials supporting the use of these devices in stage D HF and supporting data available are from observational studies. Each section in this article details the specific nuances related to each of these devices.

INTRA-AORTIC BALLOON PUMP

The intra-aortic balloon pump (IABP) is among the oldest available percutaneous TMCS options that was first described in the 1960s. It is the most commonly used TMCS device as interventional cardiologists are most familiar with it. It consists of a helium inflated balloon that is positioned in the descending aorta and pneumatically counterpulsed during diastole and actively deflated in systole (**Fig. 3**).

Hemodynamic Effects

The IABP provides a small increase in cardiac output by 0.5 L/min when dealing with cardiogenic shock. However, its hemodynamic effects are helpful in patients with stage D HF with cardiogenic shock because it decreases afterload and helps decrease the LV end-diastolic pressure (LVEDP). Balloon inflation occurs at the onset of diastole, leading to improved

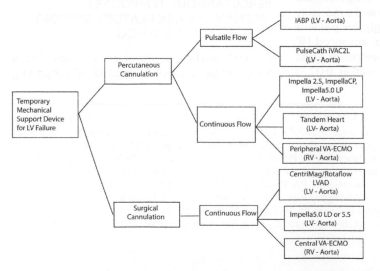

Fig. 2. Devices available for left ventricular TMCS. IABP, intra-aortic balloon pump; LP, left percutaneous. LA, left atrium; LV, left ventricle; RA, right atrium; VA-ECMO, veno-arterial extracorporeal membrane oxygenation.

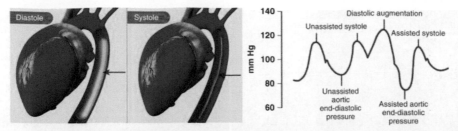

Fig. 3. The intra-aortic balloon pump located in the descending aorta is inflated during diastole and deflated during systole. Aortic pressure tracing during 1:2 counterpulsation. The first 2 beats have unassisted systole, followed by increase in peak aortic pressure with balloon inflation in diastole. Balloon deflation before systole decreases ventricular afterload. (*From* Aaronson KD, Pagani FD. Mechanical Circulatory Support. Braunwald's Heart Disease: A Textbook of Cardiovascular Medicine 2019; 568-579.; with permission.)

coronary perfusion and myocardial oxygen delivery. Balloon deflation occurs immediately before the onset of systole, leading to a decrease in systemic vascular resistance, lowering LVEDP and decreasing severity of mitral regurgitation.

Technical Considerations

An IABP can be inserted via femoral access or axillary access using a double lumen, 7.5F to 8.0F arterial sheath attached to a balloon. One lumen connects to a pump that inflates the balloon and the second allows guidewire insertion and for transducing the aortic pressure. Insertion via an axillary approach allows for ambulation while awaiting a durable LVAD or HT.[5] Under fluoroscopic guidance, the balloon is positioned immediately distal to the left subclavian artery. Helium is used for balloon inflation owing to its low viscosity, allowing rapid transfer in and out of the balloon, and because it absorbs rapidly into the blood in case of an accidental rupture of the balloon.

Because improper balloon positioning can lead to occlusion of the subclavian artery or bilateral renal arteries, fluoroscopic confirmation of device position should be obtained after insertion and daily with chest radiographs. The distal tip of the balloon, marked with a radiopaque marker, should be positioned 1 to 2 cm distal to the left subclavian artery (second to third left intercostal space; **Fig. 4**). The carina provides another useful radiographic marker to confirm positioning on chest radiographs, with studies suggesting placement of the IABP tip 2 cm above the carina.[6]

Management

A key factor that ensures deriving maximal benefit from an IABP is appropriate timing of balloon inflation and deflation. A display console attached to the device provides continuous waveform of the pressure tracing with continuous electrocardiogram (EKG) monitoring. An arterial pressure waveform is obtained from the arterial lumen of the catheter. The device can be set to time balloon counterpulsation to the EKG tracing (most commonly used) or can be based on the arterial pressure waveform. If set to EKG triggering, the balloon inflates at the middle of the T wave on the surface EKG and deflation is timed to the peak of the R-wave of the surface EKG.

Inflation of the balloon should occur on the dicrotic notch of the arterial waveform and deflation should occur just before systole. **Fig. 5** shows pressure waveforms with early and late inflation and deflation. Early inflation of the balloon can result in premature closure

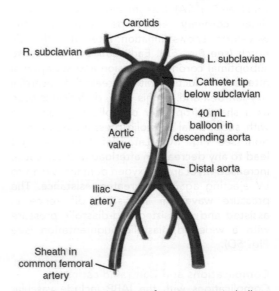

Fig. 4. Proper positioning of an intra-aortic balloon pump. The catheter tip should be below the subclavian artery, in the second or third intercostal space or at the level of the carina. (*From* Ragosta M. Textbook of clinical hemodynamics. Philadelphia: Saunders/Elsevier; 2008; with permission.)

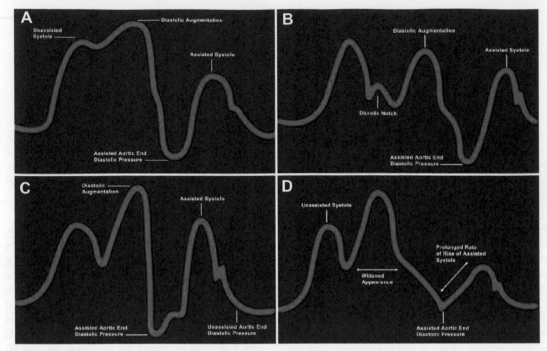

Fig. 5. IABP waveforms owing to mistimed balloon counterpulsation. (*A*) Early inflation. (*B*) Late inflation. (*C*) Early deflation. (*D*) Late deflation. (*From* Krishna M, Zacharowski K. Principles of intra-aortic balloon pump counterpulsation, Contin Educ Anaesth Crit Care Pain 2009; 9 (1): 24-28; with permission.)

of the aortic valve, causing increased afterload and myocardial oxygen demand. In this case, inflation occurs before the dicrotic notch and diastolic augmentation can encroach onto systole (see **Fig. 5**A). Late inflation leads to suboptimal coronary artery perfusion and the waveform shows inflation after the dicrotic notch (see **Fig. 5**B). Early deflation can cause suboptimal coronary perfusion and suboptimal afterload reduction with increased myocardial oxygen demand. In this case, deflation is seen as a sharp drop after diastolic augmentation with suboptimal diastolic pressure augmentation (see **Fig. 5**C). Late deflation does not lead to any decrease in afterload and can cause increased myocardial oxygen demand owing to LV ejecting against a greater resistance. The pressure waveform shows no difference in assisted and unassisted end-diastolic pressure with a widened diastolic augmentation (see **Fig. 5**D).

Complications and Contraindications

Complications with the IABP include vascular complications, such as bleeding, stroke, limb ischemia, or vascular trauma with resultant bowel or renal ischemia. Other complications include infections or thrombocytopenia from platelet deposition on the IABP membrane or

with heparin use. Contraindication to the use of an IABP includes severe aortic regurgitation as with diastolic balloon inflation, the regurgitant volume increases. Peripheral arterial disease increases the risk for vascular complications from the device, including limb ischemia.

Clinical Data

In an analysis of the INTERMACS registry examining use of an IABP before LVAD implantation by DeVore and colleagues,[7] an IABP was used in 18% of patients undergoing LVAD implantation. IABP use correlated with markers of more severe disease, including worse renal and liver function. Yet, in a propensity-matched analysis the incidence of death, postoperative right ventricular failure, renal and hepatic dysfunction was no different in patients receiving an IABP before LVAD compared with those who did not, suggesting possible risk mitigation with use of an IABP.[7] Similarly, among 88 HT candidates, in a single-center study, Tanaka and colleagues[8] described their experience with axillary–subclavian IABP. Overall, 80 patients (93.4%) were successfully bridged to definitive therapy with no mortality related to the device. The device-related complication rate was 7.9% and 95.5% patients were ambulatory.[8]

IMPELLA

The Impella series of devices (Abiomed, Danvers, MA) are continuous flow, microaxial pumps with propellers at the tips of the catheters that are positioned across the aortic valve. Based on the Archimedes screw principle, they deliver blood from the LV into the aorta by creating negative pressure at the propeller tip, which draws blood into the inlet and through the cannula (Fig. 6).

Hemodynamic Effects

Impella pumps unload the LV directly, leading to a decrease in the LVEDP and decreasing myocardial oxygen consumption. By diverting blood into the aorta, it increases forward flow improving the systemic mean arterial blood pressure (Fig. 7). These pumps provide cardiac output augmentation ranging from 2.5 L/min (Impella 2.5), 3.0 to 4.0 L/min (Impella CP), 5.0 L/min (Impella 5.0 LP and LD), and up to 6 L/min (Impella 5.5).

Technical Considerations

Impella pumps are designed to be placed via the femoral artery. The smaller 12F Impella 2.5 and 14F Impella CP can be placed percutaneously. However, larger 21F Impella 5.0 LP and 23F Impella 5.5, require a surgical cut down. The Impella 5.0 LD is designed to be inserted via open sternotomy. Impella devices consist of a pigtail catheter that is inserted in a retrograde fashion across the aortic valve with its distal end sitting in the LV and an outlet in the proximal aorta. The pigtail is connected to a 12F to 23F cannula that contains the motor housing. The only exceptions to this design are the

Impella 5.5 and 5.0 LD, which do not have a pigtail end.

Distal to the motor housing is the outlet where blood is ejected into the aorta and distal to the outlet is the differential pressure sensor that assists with the device's position detection. The Impella is then connected to an extracorporeal controller system that helps regulate function and has 9 different speed settings (P0–P8) for the propeller. The controller also houses a purge system that infuses 5% dextrose and heparin through the Impella to minimize clotting and forms a hydraulic shield that prevents blood from migrating into the motor housing (see Fig. 6).

Management

When perfectly positioned, the inlet area of the device is approximately 3.5 cm below the aortic valve and the outlet area is in the aorta. The controller will show an aortic placement signal waveform and a pulsatile current waveform. A severely dysfunctional LV may not be able to generate a significant pressure gradient across the aortic valve, leading to a dampened placement signal and motor current waveforms. In this case, positioning should be confirmed with an echocardiogram or under fluoroscopy.

If the device abuts the anterior mitral valve leaflet, it can cause functional mitral stenosis, mitral regurgitation, or hemolysis. Accordingly, hemodynamics suggesting inadequate left ventricular unloading should prompt an ascertainment of the device position.

Additional alarms related to the device include the suction alarm. This alarm can trigger if there is inadequate preload as with right ventricular dysfunction, hypovolemia, or profound

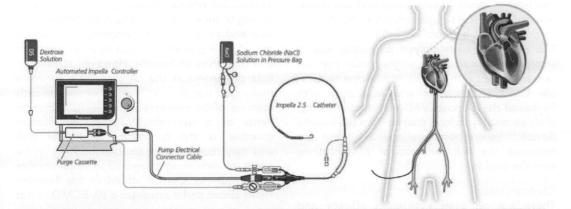

Fig. 6. Standard configuration of the Impella. (*From* Allender JE, Reed BN, Foster JL et al. Pharmacologic Considerations in the Management of Patients Receiving Left Ventricular Percutaneous Mechanical Circulatory Support. Pharmacotherapy 2017; 37(10):1272-1283; with permission.)

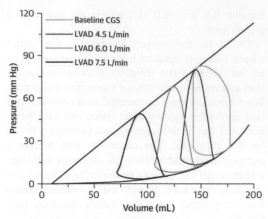

Fig. 7. Pressure–volume curve with LV to aorta assist device such as the Impella. With increased unloading, the LVEDP decreases and there is increased uncoupling of the aortic and peak left ventricular pressure generation. CGS, cardiogenic shock. (*Adapted from* Burkhoff D, Sayer G, Doshi D et al. Hemodynamic of Mechanical Circulatory Support. JACC, 2015 Dec;66(23):2663-2674; with permission.)

vasodilation, such as with sepsis. It can also occur if the device is improperly positioned and abuts into the LV. Other causes for a suction alarm include a clot in the device or a high afterload. Troubleshooting a suction alarm should involve decreasing the propeller speed, checking the volume status, and ensuring cannula is appropriately positioned.

Finally, anticoagulation is mandatory with Impella devices with an activated clotting time of greater than 250 seconds at placement and 160 to 180 seconds thereafter.

Complications and Contraindications

Hemolysis owing to mechanical shearing of red blood cells is common.[9] Persistent hemolysis can lead to acute kidney injury and worsening anemia. It can also suggest improper positioning or presence of a thrombus within the cannula. The incidence of hemolysis is greater with a smaller cannula size. In a single-center case series, treatment with Impella as a bridge to durable LVAD implantation was associated with increased risk of post-LVAD aortic insufficiency, likely secondary to local trauma from the Impella device.[10] Severe peripheral arterial disease also increases the risk for vascular complications with the device.

Clinical Data

There are no trials evaluating efficacy and safety of Impella in patients with stage D HF as a bridge to advanced therapies and evidence is limited to observational studies. Seese

and colleagues[11] evaluated the use of a surgically implanted Impella 5.0 as a bridge to transplantation among adult HT recipients in the United Network for Organ Sharing Registry. A total of 236 patients listed for a transplant were supported with an Impella 5.0. The rate of removal from the waitlist owing to clinical deterioration or death was 20%, with other patients being successfully bridged to a transplant or a durable LVAD, or had myocardial recovery. The median time on support was 13 days and 90.3% patients survived 1 year after transplantation with infrequent post-transplant complications.[11]

TandemHeart

The TandemHeart device is an extracorporeal, centrifugal continuous flow pump that diverts blood from the LA and bypasses the LV, thereby unloading it; it subsequently returns flow into the femoral artery. Accordingly, both the pump and native LV contribute flow to the aorta simultaneously or work in tandem (**Fig. 8**). It consists of a 21F venous cannula positioned in the LA via trans-septal access through the femoral vein and a 15F to 19F arterial cannula positioned in the femoral artery.

Hemodynamic Effects

TandemHeart decreases the LVEDP by venting the LA and decreases cardiac workload and myocardial oxygen demand. This may be partially offset by an increased afterload from the retrograde aortic blood flow toward the root.[12] The TandemHeart cardiac output augmentation is similar to the Impella 5.0 device at up to 5/min. It increases cardiac output and mean arterial pressure (see **Fig. 8B**).

Technical Considerations

Owing to the requirement for trans-septal puncture and placement of a large-bore cannula in the LA, this procedure requires more expertise and time than an Impella. However, stable cannula placement in the LA may allow for more prolonged use than an Impella, where the catheter tip often interacts with structural components of a dynamic LV (papillary muscles, chordae, or the contracting ventricular wall) and may require more trouble shooting. In the event of increasing oxygenation requirements, an oxygenator can be added to the Tandem-Heart circuit and it simulates a VA-ECMO circuit.

Management

Device positioning for the TandemHeart is vital because migration of the cannula into the RA

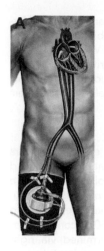

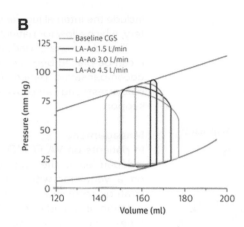

Fig. 8. (A) Tandem Heart. (B) Pressure–volume loop with LA to aorta assist devices. With increasing flow support, the LVEDP decreases, the LV end-systolic volume increases, and the LV stroke volume decreases. Ao, aorta; CGS, cardiogenic shock. (Courtesy of CardiacAssist Inc. dba Tandem-Life, Pittsburgh, PA with permission; and Adapted from Burkhoff D, Sayer G, Doshi D et al. Hemodynamic of Mechanical Circulatory Support. JACC, 2015 Dec;66(23):2663-2674; with permission.)

can create a right-to-left shunt and cause hypoxia. Migration too deep into the LA can lead to perforation and tamponade. Care must be taken to prevent the cannula from dislodging during patient movement.

Flow support provided by the device depends on adequate preload, low afterload, cannula size, and cannula position. Support is initiated at 5500 revolutions per minute and increased by 250 to 500 revolutions per minute until no further increase is noted. Low-flow alarms displayed on the console can be secondary to low preload from severe right ventricle (RV) dysfunction, hypovolemia, or tamponade; from elevated afterload; or from arrhythmias or owing to kinking of the cannula. Similar to an Impella, anticoagulation is mandatory and an activated clotting time of about 300 seconds is typically required.[13]

Complications and Contraindications

Complications with the TandemHeart are similar to other percutaneous devices and include vascular complications, such as limb ischemia, vascular injury and bleeding. Complications related to trans-septal access include cardiac tamponade. Other possible complications include air or thromboembolism and hemolysis. Cannula migration into the RA can cause right to-left-shunting and hypoxia.

Clinical Data

One small trial comparing use of the Tandem-Heart with an IABP in cardiogenic shock showed improved hemodynamic and metabolic outcomes with the TandemHeart, but without a survival benefit.[14] Smith and colleagues[15] reported outcomes in 55 patients with cardiogenic shock undergoing TandemHeart placement. The

device led to hemodynamic improvement and 51% patients were successfully bridged to LVAD or surgery. Device-related complications were noted in 9 patients (16.4%).

VENOARTERIAL EXTRA CORPOREAL MEMBRANE OXYGENATION

The ECMO technology has been in existence for nearly 7 decades and a VA-ECMO circuit provides full hemodynamic and respiratory support by oxygenating blood diverted from a systemic vein and subsequently delivering this oxygenated blood into a systemic artery (**Fig. 9**). The circuit can be deployed peripherally or centrally. This section details peripheral VA-ECMO.

Hemodynamic Effects

VA-ECMO decreases preload by diverting venous blood flow and decreases wall tension. However, its hemodynamic effects on the LV are somewhat deleterious because it may increase afterload and left ventricular workload as the blood returns to the arterial system.[12] It provides up to 4 to 6 L/min of continuous flow and the addition of an oxygenator provides full respiratory support (**Fig. 10**).

Technical Considerations

Access for peripheral VA-ECMO consists of a 21F venous cannula and a 15F to 19F arterial cannula. Routine use of antegrade perfusion cannulation to prevent limb ischemia is recommended.[16] The venous cannula drains deoxygenated blood through a centrifugal pump into a membrane oxygenator, where gas exchange takes place. Oxygenated blood is then returned through an arterial cannula. Typical cannulation sites include the femoral vein and femoral artery. Alternate sites

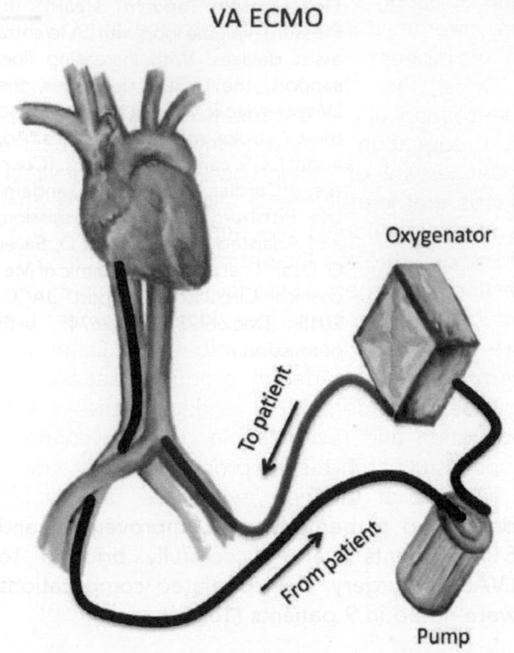

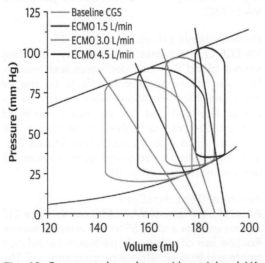

VA ECMO

Oxygenator

To patient

From patient

Pump

Fig. 9. Circuit in peripheral VA-ECMO. (*From* Foong TW, Ramanathan K, Man Chan KK et al. Extracorporeal Membrane Oxygenation During Adult Noncardiac Surgery and Perioperative Emergencies: A Narrative Review. J Cardiothorac Vasc Anesth. 2020 Jan21; 21053-0770(20)30086-0; with permission.)

Fig. 10. Pressure–volume loop with peripheral VA-ECMO. Increasing flow is associated with an increase in the LVEDP, a decrease in LV stroke volume, and an increase in the effective arterial elastance. (*Adapted from* Burkhoff D, Sayer G, Doshi D et al. Hemodynamic of Mechanical Circulatory Support. JACC, 2015 Dec;66(23):2663-2674. with permission.)

include the internal jugular vein and the axillary artery, which allow for patient mobilization.

The advantage of peripheral VA-ECMO is that it can be placed bedside in a critically ill, acutely decompensating patient (including during cardiac arrest) and can provide rapid hemodynamic support.

Management

In patients on VA-ECMO, gas exchange occurs independent of the lung, but patients are placed on a ventilator with a low-volume protective strategy to maintain lung compliance. Anticoagulation is mandatory with activated clotting times ranging from 180 to 250 seconds. Adequacy of oxygenation is determined via right radial arterial blood gases because the right subclavian is the most distal branch relative to the circuit allowing for early detection of possible north–south syndrome (described elsewhere in this article). A perfusionist is required to manage the circuit, unlike other TMCS devices.

In patients with severe LV dysfunction, support with peripheral VA-ECMO can lead to the LV being bypassed entirely causing progressive LV and LA dilatation with stagnation of blood leading to pulmonary edema (ECMO lung) and the formation of thrombi. Therefore, in patients with cardiogenic shock being bridged to durable LVAD or HT therapy, the LV may need to be unloaded by using either an IABP, an Impella (called ECPELLA), or a TandemHeart.[17] The use of these devices or surgical vent of the LV has demonstrated improved hemodynamics and survival in some patients.[18]

With recovery of the native heart, increasing circulation from the native heart flowing through congested lungs results in flow competition in the aorta between deoxygenated blood delivered from the native heart and oxygenated blood from the extracorporeal circuit leading to "north–south" syndrome (**Fig. 11**).[19] This syndrome results in deoxygenated blood being supplied to the upper one-half of the body. Measures to correct this condition include the use of an LV vent to decrease the LV end-diastolic pressure and treat ECMO lung or addition of another cannula into the circuit to send oxygenated blood (ie, a variable air volume circuit with the addition of an internal jugular cannula).

Complications and Contraindications

Complications related to peripheral VA-ECMO include vascular complications, such as, bleeding, vascular injury, infections, and limb ischemia. Other complications include bleeding from use

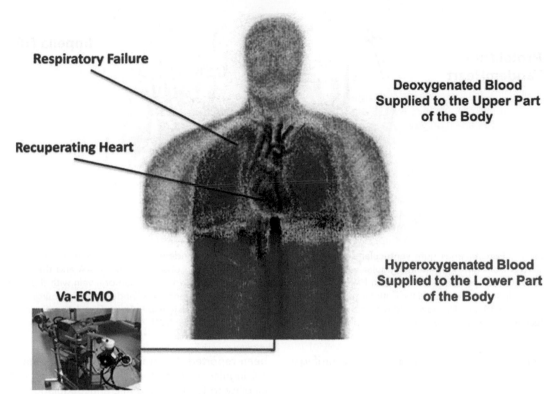

Respiratory Failure

Deoxygenated Blood
Supplied to the Upper Part
of the Body

Recuperating Heart

Hyperoxygenated Blood
Supplied to the Lower Part
of the Body

Va-ECMO

Fig. 11. North South or Harlequin syndrome on peripheral VA-ECMO. (*From* Lotz C, Ritter O and Mullenbach RM. Assisted Beating of the Ischemic Heart. Circulation 2014;130:1095-1104; with permission.)

of systemic anticoagulation and thromboembolic complications. Severe aortic insufficiency may worsen on peripheral VA-ECMO and mandate use of a LV vent.

Clinical Data

VA-ECMO can be used as a bridge to HT or durable LVAD in patients with stage D HF. Case series have reported its use for refractory cardiogenic shock with a variety of etiologies. Survival among patients on VA-ECMO is modest with an in-hospital mortality of up to 60% and a 6-month survival rate of 30%.[20,21] The underlying diagnosis is a key factor in guiding outcomes on VA-ECMO with reversible causes of myocardial injury such as fulminant myocarditis having a better survival. Another key factor that determines outcomes on VA-ECMO is the presence of multiorgan dysfunction. This factor highlights importance of appropriate timing with use of VA-ECMO before the onset of significant endorgan dysfunction.[22]

PulseCath iVAC2L

The PulseCath is a single-lumen catheter with a bidirectional valve positioned in the ascending

aorta. The catheter tip is positioned in the LV and, in synchronization with the EKG, the catheter initially aspirates blood from the LV and then ejects it into the ascending aorta via the same valve. Therefore, this microaxial flow pump allows for pulsatile forward flow and can achieve a 2 L/min augmentation of the cardiac output. An additional highlight is that the catheter has an extracorporeal pump that is powered by an IABP. This factor has made this device an attractive option for rapid use in the cardiac catheterization laboratory. The PulseCath obtained Conformite Europeenne (CE) approval and is available for use in Europe and India, primarily for supported PCI use, but also as a bridge to decision/LVAD.[23] The device is not currently approved for use in the United States.

PERCUTANEOUS TEMPORARY MECHANICAL CIRCULATORY SUPPORT FOR THE RIGHT VENTRICLE

ProtekDuo

PROTEK Duo (Cardiac Assist Inc., Pittsburgh, PA) cannula is a dual-lumen, coaxial cannula positioned via the internal jugular vein with its distal tip in the pulmonary artery (PA) and

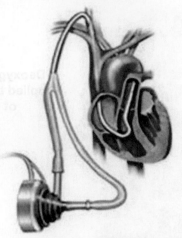
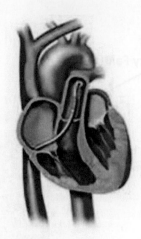

ProtekDuo TandemHeart

Impella RP

Fig. 12. Percutaneous right ventricular support devices. (1) ProtekDuo TandemHeart: a dual lumen cannula is inserted from the right internal jugular vein with the proximal inflow lumen positioned in the RA and the distal outflow lumen positioned in the main PA. (2) Impella RP: a catheter is inserted via the femoral vein with the inlet in the inferior vena cava and the outlet into the PA. (*Courtesy of* CardiacAssist Inc. dba TandemLife, Pittsburgh, PA, and Abiomed, Inc. Danvers, MA; with permission, and *From* Cowger J, Goldstein DJ. Acute Circulatory Support. Mechanical Circulatory Support: A Companion to Braunwald's Heart Disease. 2020; 41-51; with permission.)

connected to an extracorporeal centrifugal pump (Fig. 12).

Hemodynamic effects
ProtekDuo decreases the RA pressure by directly venting it and transferring blood into the PA. It increases the mean PA pressure and, by increasing preload to the LV, it increases the LV end-diastolic pressure. It can augment cardiac output by 2 to 4 L/min.

Technical considerations
The device is composed of a dual-lumen 29F to 31F catheter that is shaped like a Swan–Ganz catheter and inserted via the internal jugular vein. One lumen serves as the inflow cannula and has a series of inflow vents positioned across the superior vena cava into the RA. The inflow cannula drains into a centrifugal pump that delivers blood back into the PA via the second lumen with a multifenestrated distal tip. Owing to the access site, it allows for patient mobilization.

Management
Use of the ProtekDuo requires systemic anticoagulation. An oxygenator can be spliced into the circuit to provide respiratory support.

Complications and contraindications
As with other percutaneous devices, complications associated include vascular complications, such as access site bleeding, infections, vascular injury and systemic bleeding. Hemolysis has also

been reported. Contraindications include internal jugular venous stenosis or thrombosis and inability to tolerate systemic anticoagulation.

Current data
Data on the ProtekDuo are limited to small studies. The largest case series comprises of a 2-center study with 17 patients.[24] The mean support duration was 10.5 ± 6.5 days with 12 LVAD recipients, 2 HT recipients, 2 patients with RV failure, and 1 patient with biventricular failure. Complications occurred in 6 patients (35%), including 3 systemic bleeds owing to anticoagulation, 1 vascular site injury, and 2 access site bleeding. Overall, 41% of these patients did not survive, consistent with poor overall prognosis for RV failure.

Impella RP
Impella RP (Abiomed Inc) is a microaxial flow catheter that delivers blood from the RA into the PA (see Fig. 12).

Hemodynamic effects
The device decreases RA pressure, increases PA pressure, and increases systemic blood pressure by increasing preload to the LV. It delivers up to 4 L/min of cardiac output.

Technical considerations
Impella RP uses a 22F impeller mounted on an 11F catheter delivered via a 23F venous peel-away sheath into the PA. Once in position, the peel-away sheath is replaced by an 11F to 23F

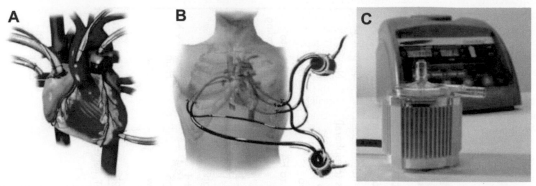

Fig. 13. CentriMag Biventricular Ventricular Assist Device cannula configuration. (*A*) Surgically implanted biventricular support. Inflow from the right atrial appendage and outflow into the main pulmonary artery for right ventricular support. Inflow from the left atrium via the right superior pulmonary vein with outflow into the ascending aorta for left ventricular support. (*B*) Cannula are connected externally to a pump (extracorporeal pump). (*C*) The centrimag device. (*From* Aaronson KD, Pagani FD. Mechanical Circulatory Support. Braunwald's Heart Disease: A Textbook of Cardiovascular Medicine 2019;568-579.)

repositioning sheath. It requires a single venous access site, which is most commonly the femoral vein.

Management
Anticoagulation is needed with Impella RP. Unlike the ProtekDuo, it cannot be used to oxygenate blood. Owing to femoral access patients cannot ambulate.

Complications and contraindications
As with ProtekDuo, complications include systemic bleeding related to the use of anticoagulation or vascular complications. Hemolysis has also been reported.

Clinical data
The RECOVER RIGHT trial prospectively evaluated Impella RP for refractory RV failure in 12

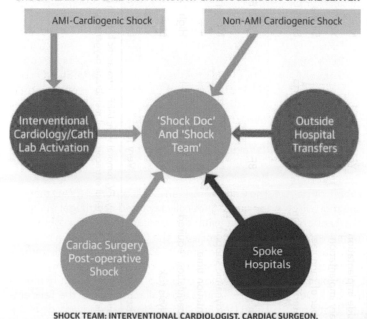

SHOCK TEAM 'ONE CALL' ACTIVATION AT CARDIOGENIC SHOCK CARE CENTER

AMI-Cardiogenic Shock

Non-AMI Cardiogenic Shock

Interventional Cardiology/Cath Lab Activation

'Shock Doc' And 'Shock Team'

Outside Hospital Transfers

Cardiac Surgery Post-operative Shock

Spoke Hospitals

SHOCK TEAM: INTERVENTIONAL CARDIOLOGIST, CARDIAC SURGEON, HEART FAILURE SPECIALIST AND CRITICAL CARE INTENSIVIST

Fig. 14. Suggested shock team composition at centers caring for patients with cardiogenic shock. (*From* Rab T. "Shock Teams" and "Shock docs". JACC 2019 Apr;73(13):1670-1672; with permission.)

Table 1
Comparison of available options for temporary mechanical left ventricular support

	IABP	Impella 2.5, CP and 5 LP	Impella 5.5	TandemHeart	VA-ECMO	CentriMag
Maximal flow (LPM)	0.5–1	2.5–5	6	5	4–6	10
Pump mechanism	Pneumatic	Axial	Axial	Centrifugal	Centrifugal	Centrifugal
Bedside implantation	Yes	No	No	No	Yes (peripheral)	No
Axillary implantation	Yes	Yes	Yes	No	No	No
Number of cannulae	Single	Single	Single	Two	Two	Two
Catheter/cannula location	Descending aorta	LV/LVOT	LV/LVOT	LA to FA	FV to FA	LA/LV to ascending aorta
Sheath size	8F	12–21F	23F	21F (FV) 15–19F (FA)	18–21F (FV) 15–19F (FA)	N/A
Hemodynamic support	Low	Moderate	High	High	High	High
Implantation time	+	++	+++	++++	+++	++++
Anticoagulation required	Very low	High	High	High	High	High
Hemolysis risk	Very low	Low	Low to moderate	Low	Low	Low
Limb ischemia risk	Very low	Low	Moderate	High	High	N/A

Abbreviations: FA, femoral artery; FV, femoral vein; IABP, intra-aortic balloon pump; LA, left atrium; LPM, liters per minute; LV, left ventricle; LVOT, left ventricular outflow tract; N/A, not applicable; VA-ECMO, veno-arterial extracorporeal membrane oxygenation.

patients with acute myocardial infarction and 18 patients after cardiac surgery. Its use was associated with a lower RA pressure and increased cardiac output. The most common complications included bleeding and hemolysis. Survival to 30 days or hospital discharge was 73%.[25]

Surgically Placed Temporary Mechanical Circulatory Support Devices

There are currently 2 continuous flow, extracorporeal centrifugal pumps placed via median sternotomy that are approved by the US Food and Drug Administration: CentriMag (Abbott Laboratories, Abbott Park, IL) and RotaFlow (MAQUET Cardiopulmonary AG, Hirrlingen, Germany). They work on the principle of generating a rotary motion with moving blades, impellers, or concentric cones and provide high flow rates with modest increases in pressure. These devices can be used to provide LV, RV, or biventricular support for up to 30 days and are pragmatic TMCS devices for bridging to durable LVAD placement or transplantation.[26,27]

Hemodynamic effects

Blood flow in a centrifugal pump is perpendicular to the rotor. The inflow cannula for LV support is placed in the LA or LV with an outflow cannula in the ascending aorta. For RV support, the inflow cannula is placed in the RA and outflow cannula in the PA. They decrease LV and RV end-diastolic pressure and decrease cardiac work and myocardial wall stress. They are capable of providing up to 10 L/min of support.

Technical considerations

CentriMag has a magnetically levitated impeller with no bearings, metal shafts, or seals (**Fig. 13**). The RotaFlow consists of a magnetically stabilized rotor levitated on a sapphire bearing. Their designs minimize friction and improve hemocompatibility. They require priming and deairing before use, but the priming volume needed for both these pumps is small, minimizing hemodilution. Both of these devices are principally designed for surgical implantation and require sternotomy for inflow cannulation in the LA or LV.

Management

Owing to the need for central access, patients supported by these devices can be mobilized. Anticoagulation is mandatory; however, these devices are forgiving of interruptions in anticoagulation.

Complications and contraindications

Complications related to these devices include bleeding related to use of systemic anticoagulation and predisposition to gastrointestinal bleeding as with durable LVADs, infections, and thromboembolism. Hemolysis can also be seen. Contraindications include the inability to tolerate systemic anticoagulation.

Current data

Evidence supporting use of these devices is limited to case series and reports.[28] Head-to-head comparisons of the 2 devices show nodifference[29]; however, RotaFlow is a less expensive option.

ROLE OF THE SHOCK TEAM AND THE ORGANIZATION OF EXPERT CENTERS

Patients with stage D HF have more comorbidities and decision-making is influenced by candidacy for advanced HF therapies. Ideally, a patient's candidacy for advanced HF therapies such as durable LVAD or HT is established before TMCS placement, and the TMCS is intended to serve as a bridge to durable therapy. If detailed advanced HF therapy evaluation has not been initiated, urgent evaluation for durable LVAD placement or HT needs to be pursued in parallel with decision-making regarding TMCS. Invasive hemodynamic assessment including RV function evaluation also informs the clinical team about the ability to successfully perform durable LVAD or HT surgery. Involvement of palliative care teams in the management of these patients should be considered.

Strategies that improve outcomes in cardiogenic shock include the implementation of a multidisciplinary shock team consisting of advanced HF cardiologists, interventional cardiologists, and cardiac surgeons with expertise in placement of percutaneous TMCS.[30] Furthermore, as with other complex procedures, a volume–outcome relationship has been established with TMCS.[31,32] These findings support the reorganization of care delivery for patients with cardiogenic shock in a spoke-and-hub fashion, similar to care delivery for trauma (**Fig. 14**).[33]

SUMMARY

A wide array of TMCS devices is available to support both the right and LV for patients in cardiogenic shock as a bridge to durable LVAD or HT. The use of these devices has increased substantially, in large part owing to the new HT allocation system combined with increased severity of illness. All devices universally increase cardiac output and the mean arterial blood pressure, but have distinct hemodynamic profiles (Table 1). The choice of a device depends on the patient's needs and the comfort of the operator and the team in managing the device. The timely institution of support by rapid identification of CS is vital to successfully bridge patients with stage D HF to definitive therapies. Multidisciplinary shock teams with an established protocol may be a key to improving outcomes.

CLINICS CARE POINTS

- Timely diagnosis is essential to improve outcomes in patients with cardiogenic shock.
- There are several temporary percutaneous devices currently available for both left and right ventricular support. There is however limited high quality evidence to guide their use.
- All temporary devices for left ventricular support increase cardiac output. With the exception of peripheral veno-arterial ECMO, all of them reduce left ventricular end diastolic pressure.
- Use of temporary percutaneous support should be guided by available resources. If unavailable, transfer to a specialized center should be considered.

DISCLOSURE

Dr E.Y. Birati reports support paid to the University of Pennsylvania from Medtronic Inc and Impulse Dynamics Ltd. The other authors have no relevant disclosures.

REFERENCES

1. Roger VL. Epidemiology of heart failure. Circ Res 2013;113(6):646–59.
2. Truby LK, Rogers JG. Advanced heart failure: epidemiology, diagnosis, and therapeutic approaches. JACC Heart Fail 2020;8(7):523–36.
3. Costanzo MR, Mills RM, Wynne J. Characteristics of "Stage D" heart failure: insights from the Acute Decompensated Heart Failure National Registry Longitudinal Module (ADHERE LM). Am Heart J 2008;155(2):339–47.
4. Fang JC, Ewald GA, Allen LA, et al. Advanced (stage D) heart failure: a statement from the Heart Failure Society of America Guidelines Committee. J Card Fail 2015;21(6):519–34.
5. Estep JD, Cordero-Reyes AM, Bhimaraj A, et al. Percutaneous placement of an intra-aortic balloon pump in the left axillary/subclavian position provides safe, ambulatory long-term support as bridge to heart transplantation. JACC Heart Fail 2013;1(5): 382–8.
6. Kim JT, Lee JR, Kim JK, et al. The carina as a useful radiographic landmark for positioning the intra-aortic balloon pump. Anesth Analg 2007;105(3): 735–8.
7. DeVore AD, Hammill BG, Patel CB, et al. Intra-aortic balloon pump use before left ventricular assist device implantation: insights from the INTERMACS Registry. ASAIO J 2018;64(2):218–24.
8. Tanaka A, Tuladhar SM, Onsager D, et al. The subclavian intraaortic balloon pump: a compelling bridge device for advanced heart failure. Ann Thorac Surg 2015;100(6):2151–7 [discussion: 2157–8].
9. Seyfarth M, Sibbing D, Bauer I, et al. A randomized clinical trial to evaluate the safety and efficacy of a percutaneous left ventricular assist device versus intra-aortic balloon pumping for treatment of cardiogenic shock caused by myocardial infarction. J Am Coll Cardiol 2008;52(19):1584–8.
10. Rao SD, Johnson B, Olia SE, et al. Treatment with Impella increases the risk of de novo aortic insufficiency post left ventricular assist device implant. J Card Fail 2020;26(10):870–5.
11. Seese L, Hickey G, Keebler ME, et al. Direct bridging to cardiac transplantation with the surgically implanted Impella 5.0 device. Clin Transplant 2020;34(3):e13818.
12. Combes A, Price S, Slutsky AS, et al. Temporary circulatory support for cardiogenic shock. Lancet 2020;396(10245):199–212.
13. Rihal CS, Naidu SS, Givertz MM, et al. 2015 SCAI/ACC/HFSA/STS Clinical Expert Consensus Statement on the Use of Percutaneous Mechanical Circulatory Support Devices in Cardiovascular Care: endorsed by the American Heart Association, the Cardiological Society of India, and Sociedad Latino Americana de Cardiologia Intervencion; Affirmation of Value by the Canadian Association of Interventional Cardiology-Association Canadienne de Cardiologie d'intervention. J Am Coll Cardiol 2015;65(19):e7–26.
14. Burkhoff D, Cohen H, Brunckhorst C, et al. A randomized multicenter clinical study to evaluate the safety and efficacy of the TandemHeart percutaneous ventricular assist device versus conventional therapy with intraaortic balloon pumping for treatment of cardiogenic shock. Am Heart J 2006;152(3):469.e1-8.
15. Smith L, Peters A, Mazimba S, et al. Outcomes of patients with cardiogenic shock treated with TandemHeart((R)) percutaneous ventricular assist device: importance of support indication and definitive therapies as determinants of prognosis. Catheter Cardiovasc Interv 2018;92(6): 1173–81.

16. Bonicolini E, Martucci G, Simons J, et al. Limb ischemia in peripheral veno-arterial extracorporeal membrane oxygenation: a narrative review of incidence, prevention, monitoring, and treatment. Crit Care 2019;23(1):266.

17. Pappalardo F, Schulte C, Pieri M, et al. Concomitant implantation of Impella((R)) on top of venoarterial extracorporeal membrane oxygenation may improve survival of patients with cardiogenic shock. Eur J Heart Fail 2017;19(3):404–12.

18. Patel SM, Lipinski J, Al-Kindi SG, et al. Simultaneous venoarterial extracorporeal membrane oxygenation and percutaneous left ventricular decompression therapy with Impella is associated with improved outcomes in refractory cardiogenic shock. ASAIO J 2019;65(1):21–8.

19. Werner NL, Coughlin M, Cooley E, et al. The University of Michigan experience with venovenoarterial hybrid mode of extracorporeal membrane oxygenation. ASAIO J 2016;62(5):578–83.

20. Batra J, Toyoda N, Goldstone AB, et al. Extracorporeal membrane oxygenation in New York State: trends, outcomes, and implications for patient selection. Circ Heart Fail 2016;9(12):e003179.

21. Takayama H, Truby L, Koekort M, et al. Clinical outcome of mechanical circulatory support for refractory cardiogenic shock in the current era. J Heart Lung Transplant 2013;32(1):106–11.

22. Keebler ME, Haddad EV, Choi CW, et al. Venoarterial extracorporeal membrane oxygenation in cardiogenic shock. JACC Heart Fail 2018;6(6):503–16.

23. den Uil CA, Daemen J, Lenzen MJ, et al. Pulsatile iVAC 2L circulatory support in high-risk percutaneous coronary intervention. EuroIntervention 2017;12(14):1689–96.

24. Ravichandran AK, Baran DA, Stelling K, et al. Outcomes with the tandem Protek duo dual-lumen percutaneous right ventricular assist device. ASAIO J 2018;64(4):570–2.

25. Anderson MB, Goldstein J, Milano C, et al. Benefits of a novel percutaneous ventricular assist device for right heart failure: the prospective RECOVER RIGHT study of the Impella RP device. J Heart Lung Transplant 2015;34(12):1549–60.

26. Takayama H, Soni L, Kalesan B, et al. Bridge-to-decision therapy with a continuous-flow external ventricular assist device in refractory cardiogenic shock of various causes. Circ Heart Fail 2014;7(5):799–806.

27. Mohite PN, Zych B, Popov AF, et al. CentriMag short-term ventricular assist as a bridge to solution in patients with advanced heart failure: use beyond 30 days. Eur J Cardiothorac Surg 2013;44(5):e310–5.

28. Nagpal AD, Singal RK, Arora RC, et al. Temporary mechanical circulatory support in cardiac critical care: a state of the art review and algorithm for device selection. Can J Cardiol 2017;33(1):110–8.

29. Palanzo DA, El-Banayosy A, Stephenson E, et al. Comparison of hemolysis between CentriMag and RotaFlow rotary blood pumps during extracorporeal membrane oxygenation. Artif Organs 2013;37(9):E162–6.

30. Tehrani BN, Truesdell AG, Sherwood MW, et al. Standardized team-based care for cardiogenic shock. J Am Coll Cardiol 2019;73(13):1659–69.

31. Barbaro RP, Odetola FO, Kidwell KM, et al. Association of hospital-level volume of extracorporeal membrane oxygenation cases and mortality. Analysis of the extracorporeal life support organization registry. Am J Respir Crit Care Med 2015;191(8):894–901.

32. Shaefi S, O'Gara B, Kociol RD, et al. Effect of cardiogenic shock hospital volume on mortality in patients with cardiogenic shock. J Am Heart Assoc 2015;4(1):e001462.

33. MacKenzie EJ, Rivara FP, Jurkovich GJ, et al. A national evaluation of the effect of trauma-center care on mortality. N Engl J Med 2006;354(4):366–78.

Large Sheath Management in Patients with Poor Peripheral Access

Amir Kaki, MD[a],*, Hemindermeet Singh, MD[b]

KEYWORDS

- Large bore access • Peripheral arterial disease • Occlusive sheath management • Lithotripsy

KEY POINTS

- Peripheral arterial disease is associated with increased vascular complications in cardiac catheterization procedures specially involving use of large bore arteriotomies.
- Insertion of large bore sheaths in patients with poor peripheral access can result in vessel occlusion and acute limb ischemia.
- Various strategies that can be used to maintain distal limb perfusion with large bore sheath in situ are described.
- Although the common femoral artery remains the access site of choice for insertion of large bore sheaths, the percutaneous axillary artery access is a safe and reliable alternative.

INTRODUCTION

The boundaries of Interventional Cardiology are actively expanding with an exponential increase in use of percutaneous catheter-based procedures involving large bore arteriotomies including transcatheter aortic valve replacement (TAVR), endovascular repair of descending and thoracic aorta, and mechanical circulatory support (MCS) implantation. Meticulous access site management is critical for safety and overall outcomes in these procedures involving the highest risk patients. Despite the evolution of device technology and increasing operator experience, vascular and bleeding complications remain a major source of perioperative morbidity and mortality especially in older patients with multiple comorbidities.[1] Also, these complications are more frequent in emergent conditions (eg, cardiogenic shock with inotropes and vasopressors), women (due to small vessel size), and patients with underlying peripheral arterial disease (PAD).

Several percutaneous mechanical circulatory support devices are increasingly used as part of contemporary management of patients with acute myocardial infarction and cardiogenic shock based on emerging data from many observational reports.[2,3] They are also indicated in patients undergoing high-risk coronary interventions.[4] Based on the amount of hemodynamic support required, operators select different percutaneous MCS devices that provide adequate circulatory support during high-risk procedures. TandemHeart (TandemLife, Pittsburg, PA) and venoarterial extracorporeal membrane oxygenation (VA-ECMO) require 2 large bore cannulas—one inserted into the vein (and into the left atrium via transseptal puncture for TandemHeart) and another into the artery. MCS devices that only require arterial access include iVAC2L (Terumo Europe, formerly Pulse-Cath) and Impella (Abiomed, Danvers, MA). The iVAC2L device uses an intra-aortic balloon pump console and requires a 19-F sheath. The Impella 2.5 and CP provide direct cardiac unloading and

[a] Division of Interventional Cardiology, Department of Medicine, Ascension St John Hospital, 22101 Moross Road, Detroit, MI 48236, USA; [b] Division of Cardiology, Department of Medicine, Mercy-Health St Vincent Medical Center, 2409 Cherry Street, Suite 100, Toledo, OH 43608, USA
* Corresponding author.
E-mail address: dramirkaki@hotmail.com

Intervent Cardiol Clin 10 (2021) 251–255
https://doi.org/10.1016/j.iccl.2020.12.003
2211-7458/21/© 2020 Elsevier Inc. All rights reserved.

antegrade continuous flow of up to 2.5 and 4 L/min, respectively, and require a single arterial access of 13 and 14 F, respectively. The perfusion of limb distal to the large sheath is important in patients receiving these devices especially when used for prolonged duration and in patients with poor peripheral access.

The common femoral artery is the access site of choice for large bore arteriotomies in most of the MCS and TAVR procedures.[5,6] The iliofemoral anatomy, however, varies among different patient population. Furthermore, presence of atherosclerosis can significantly alter the vessel caliber and integrity of its endothelium. PAD is frequently encountered in patients with complex coronary artery disease and aortic stenosis.[7,8] The rate of vascular complications with large bore access in patients with PAD and small-caliber iliofemoral arteries is as high as 17%.[9,10] In some patients, femoral vascular access is prohibitive for large bore cannulation, as there is increased risk of complete occlusion, dissection, and perforation. In these situations, alternative arterial access sites such as the axillary artery, subclavian artery, transcaval, and direct transapical approaches may be contemplated.[11–14] Thus, thorough preoperative assessment of iliofemoral anatomy is imperative before implantation of any large bore sheath.

MANAGEMENT OF OCCLUSIVE LARGE BORE SHEATH

Insertion of large bore sheaths in patients with PAD can result in complete vessel occlusion and acute limb ischemia threatening its viability. It is therefore important to maintain adequate distal perfusion, which can be achieved with several different interventions.[15] First, after insertion of a large sheath in common femoral artery, angiogram should be obtained from the contralateral side to assess vessel patency and distal perfusion (Fig. 1). If the limb perfusion is compromised, it may be necessary to establish flow distally by an external or internal bypass circuit.

Peel-Away Sheath
The percutaneous ventricular assist device (Impella) comes with a specially designed two-step peel-away sheath with a tapered shaft (14-F base to 9-F tip) that allows for adequate blood flow even in smaller-caliber iliofemoral arterial vessels. In case of an occlusive sheath, peeling away the 14-F introducer sheath leaves the Impella with the smaller 9-F repositioning sheath, which may be sufficient to restore limb

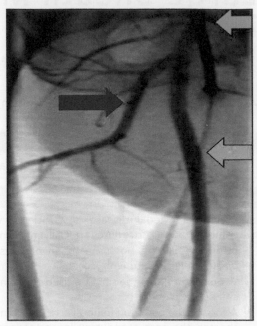

Fig. 1. Right femoral angiogram using the contralateral femoral access showing the large bore sheath (*green arrow*), superficial femoral artery (*yellow arrow*), and profunda femoral artery (*red arrow*).

perfusion. One potential complication of this technique is catheter migration while peeling away the sheath. To minimize this complication, one operator should stabilize the Impella, whereas the other operator peels away the external sheath. The repositioning sheath can then be readvanced through the arteriotomy site. This maneuver, however, may lead to increased bleeding around the access site as the sheath size is tapered down.

External Contralateral Bypass Circuit
In this technique, the ipsilateral superficial femoral artery (SFA) is accessed with a 4-F or 6-F micropuncture sheath in an antegrade fashion. Contralateral common femoral artery access is then obtained with a 6-F sheath. The side arm of the contralateral sheath is then connected to the side arm of the ipsilateral antegrade sheath using a male-to-male connector. The result is an external femoral-femoral bypass whereby blood flows from the contralateral 6-F sheath through the side arm into the side arm of the ipsilateral 4- to 6-F antegrade sheath down the ischemic limb providing adequate perfusion (Fig. 2). This antegrade access can be secured preemptively in situations where chances of common femoral artery occlusion are high, for example, in VA-ECMO. The target

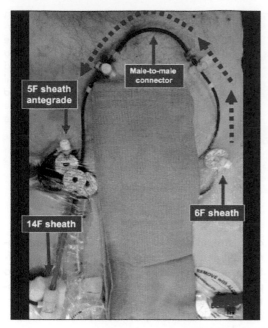

Fig. 2. An external contralateral conduit created from the contralateral femoral artery. A 6-F sheath was used in the left common femoral artery and a 4-F antegrade sheath is inserted in right superficial femoral artery beyond the large bore access site. The side arm of the "donor/mother" sheath on left side and "recipient/daughter" on right were connected using a male-to-male connector to create flow from the left to right femoral artery (*dotted arrows*).

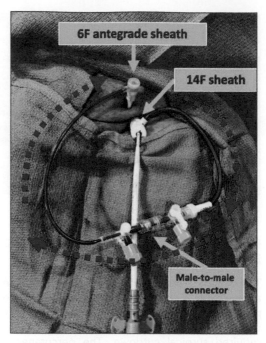

Fig. 3. An external ipsilateral bypass created from the left common femoral artery. A 6-F sheath is used to access the left common femoral artery in an antegrade puncture position distal to the large sheath. The side arm of the 6-F sheath was connected to the large sheath using a male-to-male connector, creating flow (*dotted arrow*).

activated clotting time (ACT) should be longer than standard to maintain the flow (range, 200–220 seconds). Also, hourly serial Doppler ultrasound assessment of the lower extremity pulsations is recommended.

External Ipsilateral Bypass Circuit
Another alternative technique to restore distal limb perfusion is to use the side arm of the large bore occlusive sheath to create an ipsilateral bypass circuit. A 4- to 6-F sheath is inserted in the ipsilateral SFA in an antegrade fashion. The side arm of the ipsilateral antegrade sheath can then be connected via a male-to-male connector to the side arm of the large bore occlusive sheath, creating an external ipsilateral bypass (Fig. 3). When using this strategy with an Impella device, the repositioning sheath must not be advanced into the Impella 14-F sheath to avoid occlusion of the side arm that is now providing perfusion.

Internal Contralateral Bypass Circuit
In patients with severe PAD, superficial femoral artery can have significant disease that precludes placement of an antegrade sheath. In such cases, an internal contralateral femoral-to-profunda bypass circuit might be an alternative option to maintain distal limb perfusion. This bypass is performed by first inserting a 7-F sheath in the contralateral common femoral artery. Through this sheath, a 5-F Internal mammary catheter is advanced and selectively engaged into the ipsilateral common iliac artery. A 0.035-inch hydrophilic wire (eg, Glidewire advantage, Terumo Interventional Systems) is then advanced through this system, past the occlusive large bore sheath, into the ipsilateral profunda femoris artery. The 5-F catheter is then exchanged for a 4-F, 45- to 55-cm long crossover sheath positioned in ipsilateral profunda. The side arm of the 7-F contralateral sheath is then connected to that of 4-F long crossover sheath using a male-to-male connector creating an internal bypass circuit whereby blood flows from the contralateral femoral artery into the ipsilateral profunda femoris artery distal to the occlusive sheath. The patient should be adequately anticoagulated with heparin for a target ACT range of 200 to 220 seconds in order to avoid circuit thrombosis.

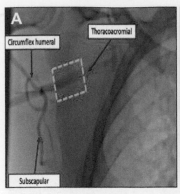
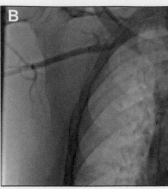

Fig. 4. Angiographic assessment and identification of the axillary artery branches to precisely define the access point that is lateral to the thoracoacromial artery and medial to the circumflex humeral and subscapular arteries (*dotted green box*) (*A*). Selective innominate contrast angiogram showing the axillary artery anatomy (*B*).

PERCUTANEOUS AXILLARY ARTERY LARGE BORE ACCESS

The axillary artery is an acceptable alternative access for large sheaths in patients with severe peripheral artery disease.[16,17] Historically, any upper extremity large bore arterial access required surgical cutdown. The percutaneous access of axially artery has recently gained popularity, as the data suggest favorable safety outcomes. In a single-center study of 48 patients who presented with cardiogenic shock or high-risk coronary interventions requiring MCS via axillary artery due to prohibitive PAD, none of the patients who died had vascular complications related to axillary access.[18] In addition, the incidence of atherosclerotic occlusion of axillary artery is noted to be lower as compared with femoral artery in PAD.[19] The caliber of the axillary artery ranges from 6 to 7 mm, which makes it suitable to accommodate sheaths with an outer diameter of up to 18F.[20] The axillary artery should be accessed between its second and third portion at the lateral border of the pectoralis minor muscle in order to avoid trauma to brachial plexus and reduce chances of pneumothorax (Fig. 4).

ACUTE LIMB ISCHEMIA

Acute limb ischemia in the setting of large bore access can be due to complete vessel occlusion (when the vessel diameter is <5 mm), arterial dissection, or thromboembolism.[1] Utilization of a femoral-femoral bypass circuit, as previously described, may prevent these complications. Close monitoring to ensure adequate limb perfusion with hourly clinical and doppler assessment of distal extremity pulses is indicated when the sheath is in place. Thromboembolism and plaque embolization are not uncommon complications. Thrombus or debris may flow downstream causing occlusion of the tibioperoneal trifurcation causing acute limb ischemia. After sheath removal, it is recommended to perform complete angiography of the arteriotomy site and runoff to the tibioperoneal trifurcation at the end of procedure to ensure distal vessel patency.

In cases where occlusion of axillary artery is anticipated with the large bore sheath, an external bypass can be created by inserting a 6-F sheath in the ipsilateral radial artery and connecting its side port to that of the large bore. Similarly, an external conduit can also be created between large bore sheath and ipsilateral brachial artery.

SUMMARY

Presence of PAD is associated with increased vascular complications, especially with use of large bore sheaths. In addition, the large bore sheaths can cause distal limb ischemia by occluding the diseased vessel. Through this article, the authors demonstrate importance of assessment for PAD before insertion of large bore sheaths. They also describe various strategies to manage occlusive sheaths for distal reperfusion and maintain limb viability, which can be used with good success rate in those who require mechanical support device of prolonged duration.

CLINICS CARE POINTS

- Peripheral arterial disease should not preclude the use of hemodynamic support in patients whom it is indicated.
- Retrograde or antegrade perfusion sheaths may help to prevent limb ischemia in patients who require large both arterial access.

- Alternative access may be considered in patients whom are not candidates for standard femoral arterial access.

DISCLOSURE

A. Kaki is a speaker and proctor for ABIOMED. The other author has no financial or proprietary interest in the subject matter of this article.

REFERENCES

1. Redfors B, Watson BM, McAndrew T, et al. Mortality, length of stay, and cost implications of procedural bleeding after percutaneous interventions using large-bore catheters. JAMA Cardiol 2017;2: 798–802.

2. Griffith BP, Anderson MB, Samuels LE, et al. The RECOVER I: a multicenter prospective study of Impella 5.0/LD for postcardiotomy circulatory support. J Thorac Cardiovasc Surg 2013;145:548–54.

3. Basir MB, Schreiber T, Dixon S, et al. Feasibility of early mechanical circulatory support in acute myocardial infarction complicated by cardiogenic shock: the Detroit Cardiogenic Shock Initiative. Catheter Cardiovasc Interv 2017;91:454–61.

4. O'Neill W, Kleiman N, Moses J, et al. A prospective, randomized clinical trial of hemodynamic support with impella 2.5 versus intra-aortic balloon pump in patients undergoing high-risk percutaneous coronary intervention. the PROTECT II Study. Circulation 2012;126:1717–27.

5. Mehta SR, Jolly SS, Cairns J, et al. Effects of radial versus femoral artery access in patients with acute coronary syndromes with or without ST-segment elevation. J Am Coll Cardiol 2012;60(24):2490–9.

6. Jolly SS, Yusuf S, Cairns J, et al. Radial versus femoral access for coronary angiography and intervention in patients with acute coronary syndromes (RIVAL): a randomised, parallel group, multicentre trial. Lancet 2011;377(9775):1409–20.

7. Gerhard-Herman MD, Gornik HL, Barrett C, et al. 2016 AHA/ACC guideline on the management of patients with lower extremity peripheral artery disease: executive summary: a report of the American College of Cardiology/American Heart Association Task Force on Clinical Practice Guidelines. J Am Coll Cardiol 2017;69(11):1465–508 [published correction appears in J Am Coll Cardiol 2017; 69(11):1520].

8. Task Force Members, Montalescot G, Sechtem U, et al. 2013 ESC guidelines on the management of stable coronary artery disease: the task force on the management of stable coronary artery disease of the European Society of Cardiology. Eur Heart J 2013;34(38):2949–3003 [published correction appears in Eur Heart J 2014;35(33):2260–1].

9. Judkins MP, Gander MP. Prevention of complications of coronary arteriography. Circulation 1974; 49:599–602.

10. Samal AK, White CJ. Percutaneous management of access site complications. Catheter Cardiovasc Interv 2002;57:12–23.

11. Walther T, Simon P, Dewey T, et al. Transapical minimally invasive aortic valve implantation: multicenter experience. Circulation 2007;116(11 suppl): I240-5.

12. Htyte N, White CJ. Vascular access for percutaneous interventions and angiography. In: Mukherjee D, Bates ER, Roffi M, et al, editors. Cardiovascular catheterization and intervention: a textbook of coronary, peripheral, and structural heart disease. 2nd edition. Boca Raton (FL): CRC Press; 2017. p. 89–112.

13. Bauernschmitt R, Schreiber C, Bleiziffer S, et al. Transcatheter aortic valve implantation through the ascending aorta: an alternative option for no-access patients. Heart Surg Forum 2009;12: E63–4.

14. Greenbaum AB, O'Neill WW, Paone G, et al. Caval-aortic access to allow transcatheter aortic valve replacement in otherwise ineligible patients: initial human experience. J Am Coll Cardiol 2014;63(25 Pt A):2795–804.

15. Kaki A, Chadi Alraes M, Kajy M, et al. Large bore occlusive sheath management. Catheter Cardiovasc Interv 2019;93:678–84.

16. Tayal R, Iftikhar H, LeSar B, et al. CT angiography analysis of axillary artery diameter versus common femoral artery diameter: implications for axillary approach for transcatheter aortic valve replacement in patients with hostile aortoiliac segment and advanced lung disease. Int J Vasc Med 2016; 2016:3610705.

17. Arnett DM, Lee JC, Harms MA, et al. Caliber and fitness of the axillary artery as a conduit for large-bore cardiovascular procedures. Catheter Cardiovasc Interv 2018;91:150–6.

18. Kaki A, Blank N, Alraies MC, et al. Axillary artery access for mechanical circulatory support devices in patients with prohibitive peripheral arterial disease presenting with cardiogenic shock. Am J Cardiol 2019;123(10):1715–21.

19. Bruschi G, Fratto P, De Marco F, et al. The trans-subclavian retrograde approach for transcatheter aortic valve replacement: single-center experience. J Thorac Cardiovasc Surg 2010;140(4):911–5.e2.

20. McBride LR, Miller LW, Naunheim KS, et al. Axillary artery insertion of an intraaortic balloon pump. Ann Thorac Surg 1989;48(6):874–5.

Alternative Access for Mechanical Circulatory Support

Amy E. Cheney, MD, James M. McCabe, MD*

KEYWORDS

- Transaxillary • Transcaval • Alternative access

KEY POINTS

- Common femoral arterial access is the de facto strategy for large-bore interventional procedures.
- The presence of significant peripheral arterial disease may preclude iliofemoral access and prompt the need for alternative percutaneous access.
- The 2 most common percutaneous alternative access options are transaxillary and transcaval approaches.
- There are advantages and disadvantages to transaxillary and transcaval access, which must be weighed in each clinical scenario.

INTRODUCTION

To date, femoral arterial access has been the standard of care for large-bore devices given vessel size and ease of management with both surgical and percutaneous techniques.[1,2] However, procedural bleeding complications are common in the setting of large-bore access and are associated with significant increases in mortality, length of stay, and health care costs.[3] Peripheral arterial disease and concomitant potential for distal limb ischemia, vessel tortuosity, and limitations related to implant durability increasingly necessitate alternative approaches to large-bore access. Earlier iterations of alternative access (typically in the setting of transcatheter aortic valve replacement [TAVR]) primarily focused on surgical intrathoracic access such as transapical and transaortic access. However, multiple analyses have shown increased morbidity and mortality in addition to increased incidence of stroke and bleeding, vascular complications, and left ventricular dysfunction.[4–6]

In addition to these disadvantages, multiple advances in transcatheter therapies have increased the feasibility of large-bore percutaneous arterial access. These advances include the continued evolution of catheter-based structural heart technologies and short-term ventricular assist devices.[7–10] Despite the growth of these technologies, access sheath sizes still typically remain greater than 10 French, which may be problematic in a population in whom peripheral arterial disease is common. When femoral access is unavailable or unattractive, alternatives to transfemoral access are critical. Thus, novel approaches to large-bore arterial access are increasingly used by contemporary interventional cardiologists and supported by contemporaneous heart teams. This article provides an overview and comparison of the 2 most common percutaneous alternative access options for large-bore sheaths: transaxillary and transcaval access.

TRANSAXILLARY ACCESS

Percutaneous access of the axillary artery has traditionally been sidestepped because of several concerns that are largely theoretic.[11,12]

Department of Internal Medicine, Division of Cardiology, University of Washington Medical Center, 1959 Northeast Pacific Street, Seattle, WA 98195-6171, USA
* Corresponding author.
E-mail address: jmmccabe@cardiology.washington.edu

Intervent Cardiol Clin 10 (2021) 257–268
https://doi.org/10.1016/j.iccl.2020.12.001
2211-7458/21/© 2020 Elsevier Inc. All rights reserved.

First, the media of the subclavian artery has a higher proportion of elastic fibers relative to the thicker media layer of the femoral artery, which consists mostly of smooth muscle cells.[13] This difference informed the concept that the subclavian and axillary arteries are more fragile than the femoral arteries, but, to date, no differences in vessel disarticulation have been observed in clinical practice. Other investigators cite concern that complication rates involving adjacent thoracic structures, such as the brachial plexus, may be higher, but, once again, there are few data to support this hypothesis. In addition, the axillary artery has for some time been misunderstood to be noncompressible, and thus access was thought only to be safely pursued by surgical cutdown enabling direct control of bleeding. Using cadaveric models, our group has shown that the proximal portion of the axillary artery may be compressed against the second rib, and clinical experience shows adequate hemostasis with manual pressure. Thus, a growing experience with large-bore, axillary arterial access has developed, showing that adequate control of the arteriotomy using percutaneous techniques is possible from implantation to final hemostasis.[14–18]

A review of axillary arterial anatomy shows that it is divided into 3 segments. The first and most proximal section is between the lateral margin of the first rib and the medial border of the pectoralis minor muscle, the second segment is deep to the pectoralis minor muscle, and the third segment is located between the lateral border of the pectoralis minor muscle and the inferior border of the teres major muscle.[16,19] Typical percutaneous axillary artery puncture occurs at the distal end of the first segment or proximal end of the second segment with the needle traversing the pectoralis minor muscle (Fig. 1).

In general, the axillary is of smaller caliber vessel than the common femoral. In a retrospective analysis of 110 computed tomography (CT) scans at a single institution, the mean diameter of the axillary artery was 6.38 mm on the right and 6.52 mm on the left.[20] An additional single-center retrospective review of 208 slightly older patients undergoing CT in anticipation of TAVR showed a mean diameter of the proximal segment of the axillary artery of 6.05 mm, which was 0.5 mm smaller than the corresponding lower extremity vessels.[19] However, a 6-mm axillary artery may still tolerate a nearly 18-French outer-diameter catheter, which is well within the typical specifications of short-term Mechanical Circulatory Support (MCS) devices and transcatheter valve systems.

A lack of obstructive atherosclerosis makes the axillary artery appealing. By CT angiogram (CTA), only 2% of patients had obstructive peripheral arterial disease of the axillary or subclavian arteries compared with 12% in iliofemoral vessels of the same population.[19] In this analysis, although diabetes and tobacco use correlated with smaller vessels, conditions known to increase calcification and atherosclerotic disease burden, such as diabetes and dialysis-dependent kidney disease, were not associated with increased calcification of the thoracic vasculature.

Preprocedural imaging is helpful in transaxillary access. This imaging comes in multiple forms, each with advantages and disadvantages. The most comprehensive imaging is high-resolution CTA. The ideal CTA window captures both axillary arteries and the ostial and proximal segments of the vertebral arteries. CTA provides information regarding vessel caliber, atherosclerosis, and angulation, particularly with the aorta. However, SCT scans necessitate contrast, require advanced planning relative to the intended procedure, and are more costly. In addition, there are 2 important considerations regarding CTAs. First, the patients are commonly asked to raise their arms above their heads during the examinations, which creates a misleading flexure or kink in the second segment of the axillary. This flexure is not fixed and furthermore is almost universally more distal than the intended point of access in the vessel.[16] Second, the venous return of contrast in this study frequently overlaps the axillary artery. Depending on the timing of the image acquisition, use of a saline chaser following contrast injection, and automated postprocessing software, there may be overlay of this venous phase filling on top of the artery, creating a false impression of significant vessel calcification. Reviewing the raw axial slices of the CT scan can easily dispel any confusion in this regard.

An alternative imaging modality is ultrasonography, which can provide caliber measurements and a sense of the atherosclerotic burden and calcification of the axillary artery. Ultrasonography does not require contrast and is less expensive than CTA but does not provide information about the subclavian arteries or the angulation of the great vessels with respect to the aorta. In addition, direct angiography of the axillary artery can be performed in advance or as part of the index procedure. Angiography provides a two-dimensional measure of vessel

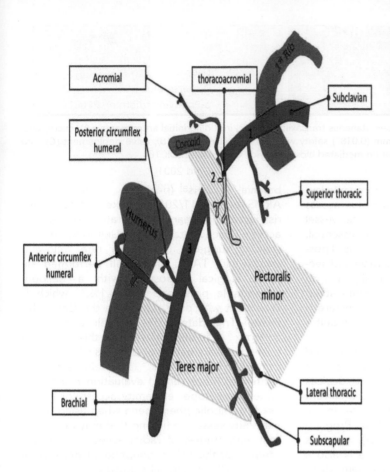

Fig. 1. The upper extremity arteries. Labels 1-3 refer to the respective axillary artery segments as defined by their relationship to Pectoralis Minor. (*From* Tai Z. Case report: "PercAx Impella": Axillary artery as an alternative access for large-bore devices. CathLab Digest 2018;26(3): with permission.)

caliber and shows obstructive plaque burden and angulation of the great vessel from the aorta. Not surprisingly, angiography is less effective at showing vessel calcification, and, if done as part of the index procedure, can make room setup more difficult if one axillary artery is more favorable than the other.

With regard to laterality of axillary arterial access, there are no convincing data to support choosing between accessing the right or left axillary artery. Regardless, multiple factors can be considered, including operator ergonomics and comfort, patient handedness, differential vessel health and caliber, patent internal mammary bypass grafts, preexisting pacemakers and defibrillators, great vessel angulation with respect to the aortic arch, risk of stroke, and, in the case of transcatheter valve implantation, coaxiality with the native annulus. None of these features are known to be absolute contraindications, although, when possible, the authors have generally tried to avoid using the axillary artery supplying the patient's dominant hand or any side with a patent internal mammary.[16] With

regard to stroke or emboli to cerebral vessels, any right axillary access necessarily crosses the right common carotid artery, whereas the left crosses the left vertebral and traverses the arch when used for technologies intended for the heart. Right axillary access also precludes use of any currently commercially available cerebral embolic protection devices. In the Axillary Registry to Monitor Safety (ARMS) multicenter registry, the primary predictor of laterality was simply operator preference, which reflects the lack of available data.[21]

Multiple articles and book chapters describe the operations of percutaneous axillary access (Fig. 2).[13,16,20,22,23] There are 2 key elements to successful percutaneous axillary access worth considering. Ultrasonography-guided access with a micropuncture system should be considered best practice given adjacent structures including the brachial plexus, lung, and axillary vein. The axillary artery runs cephalad to the vein when moving laterally with the ultrasound probe. In scenarios where the vein appears to override the artery, the operator should move

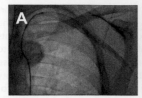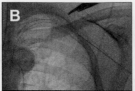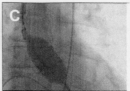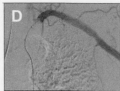

Fig. 2. Fluoroscopic images from a percutaneous transaxillary TAVR, including initial angiography (*A*), micropuncture needle stick parallel to a 0.46-mm (0.018″) safety wire in the axillary artery (*B*), valve deployment (*C*), and completion angiography following suture-mediated closure device deployment (*D*).

more laterally, away from the sternum and clavicle. Once an acceptable position for access has been established, puncturing the vessel with a shallow-angle needle stick is essential. There are bony structures both anterior and posterior to the axillary artery (the clavicle and second rib, respectively) that can easily kink an access sheath following a puncture with a steep entry angle. At our center, the skin puncture is usually close to the inferior aspect of the deltopectoral groove.

The authors routinely use suture-mediated closure devices in the axillary artery, and case reports using other vascular closure devices have been published.[24,25] Most of the current experience with vascular closure devices in the axillary artery is with the Perclose Proglide (Abbott Vascular, Santa Clara, CA), which is effective. However, manual pressure is also a feasible mechanism for establishing hemostasis of the axillary artery. The authors have successfully shown this both in perfused cadaveric specimens and in clinical practice. In addition, the results of a cohort of 46 patients who underwent a 50-cm³ intra-aortic balloon pump was recently published. Twenty-nine out of 46 (63%) achieved axillary artery homeostasis via manual compression with a median compression time of 20 minutes (range, 5–60 minutes). There were no major vascular or bleeding complications. The remainder of the patients had catheter removal with a variety of techniques, including closure device (Angio-Seal) and balloon tamponade.[26]

The typical axillary artery access point is extrathoracic, and at the distal end of the first segment or proximal end of the second segment. If bleeding complications occur from this location, they do not result in occult accumulation or hemothorax but in hematoma or ecchymosis (**Fig. 3**). Nevertheless, completion angiography following axillary artery hemostasis is strongly recommended following closure because most reported neurologic complaints seem to develop late, presumably from localized hematoma externally compressing the

brachial plexus (personal communication, ARMS registry, 11/2018). Stroke is an additional risk factor that bears consideration with axillary access. Recent data from the United States TVT registry suggests the stroke rate following transaxillary TAVR (almost all performed via open surgical exposure) with a balloon-expandable prosthesis was 6.1%,[27] which is consistent with prior data from the CoreValve Pivotal Trial data (6.5% in their transaxillary cohort).[28] It is unclear whether this is related to the high-risk nature of patients who are presumably vasculopaths, ascertainment bias related to more careful evaluation of patients undergoing upper extremity access, or higher risk for embolic phenomena when using upper extremity vessels, a finding that may be consistent with studies of radial access.[25,29] It also seems that this risk is independent of percutaneous or direct surgical exposure.[27]

Although the worldwide experience for large-bore percutaneous axillary artery access remains small, multiple successful case reports and series exist.[13,16,19,29–37]

More recently, the Axillary Registry to Monitor Safety (ARMS) was completed. ARMS was a prospective multicenter registry of percutaneous upper extremity access for MCS devices. This registry, implemented across 10 institutions in the United States, represents the largest prospective series to date. It was developed to evaluate the procedural and short-term safety of percutaneous axillary access for Impella devices (Abiomed, Danvers, MA) and intra-aortic balloons pumps. Formal publication of the completed dataset is expected soon and an interim analysis of the first 80 patients has been presented, suggesting very favorable bleeding and complication rates and no cases of ischemic upper extremity or significant neurologic injury.[21] However, there are not yet any time series data regarding the rate of complications for indwelling transaxillary devices, although it does stand to reason that the rate of vascular complications may be higher for indwelling devices compared with

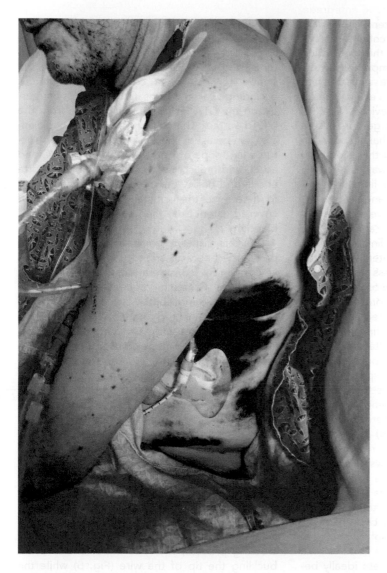

Fig. 3. Ecchymoses along the lateral flank of a patient who developed internal bleeding on day 17 following percutaneously placement of an Impella CP (Abiomed, Danvers, MA) in the axillary artery.

those that use the axillary artery for just a brief period.

THE CAVAL-AORTIC (TRANSCAVAL) APPROACH

Transcaval (caval-aortic) access was first pioneered in 2010 at the National Institutes of Health (NIH) as a proposed solution for delivery issues using large-bore devices.[38] After concept refinement and testing in animals, the first-in-human TAVR was performed in 2013 by Greenbaum and colleagues.[39]

The primary data for transcaval access are derived from a prospective, independently adjudicated, multicenter registry of 100 patients undergoing TAVR. These patients were deemed either ineligible or at high risk for femoral arterial access.[40] This registry showed a 99% TAVR success rate, 7% rate of Valve Academic Research Consortium-2 (VARC-2) life-threatening bleeding, and 13% rate of major vascular complications during the procedure. There were no subsequent vascular complications between discharge and 30 days. However, these data should be interpreted in the context of 2 important features. First, there were no roll-in patients in this registry, which generally represents the earliest possible experience in the world. Second, it is essential to recall that transfemoral large-bore access carries an appreciable bleeding risk. Using a comparable device, the transfemoral TAVR arm of the The Placement of Aortic Transcatheter Valve Trial (PARTNER) II trial showed a 6.7% life-threatening bleeding rate in an overall lower-risk cohort.[41] More recently, the 1-year results of this population were published, including a comprehensive CT analysis, and, remarkably, there were no late bleeding or vascular complication events related to the access point or closure device.[42,43]

Transcaval access facilitates large-bore access by creating a sheath-mediated channel between the inferior vena cava (IVC) and the abdominal aorta, where the arterial pathway is typically much larger, thereby bypassing iliofemoral arteries in favor of the femoral and iliac veins. Although not immediately intuitive as a mechanism for large-bore access, this approach has proved to be highly safe in clinical practice, albeit in a limited number of centers worldwide.

Conceptually, transcaval access uses 2 ideas that are not routinely considered or used during other interventional cardiology procedures: (1) that electrified wires can be steered across multiple tissue planes, thereby creating a connection between the IVC and aorta even when these vessels are not directly in contact; and (2) that an intact retroperitoneal space has an intrinsic pressure that supersedes the IVC pressure, thus rendering the IVC venotomy site a functional drain for the retroperitoneum and obviating (in fact, discouraging) IVC closure. This latter point is why significant right ventricular dysfunction and biventricular systolic dysfunction are relative contraindications to transcaval access, because both may increase IVC pressure, although in practice it is likely the transient high-output fistula from the aorta to cava following closure that can exacerbate right ventricular dysfunction.

The process of transcaval access ideally begins with careful preprocedural imaging. In this case, CTA of the abdomen and pelvis is the ideal form of preprocedural imaging, although angiograms alone can be used if required once a transcaval program is established. Specific to transcaval access planning, there are 2 interrelated questions to address when reviewing the CTA: is there a calcium-free zone in the abdominal aorta conducive to transcaval access, and, if so, where? This topic has been judiciously addressed in the literature.[44] Briefly, a calcium-free area needs to be identified along the aortic wall facing the IVC that is neither so low as to be close to the aortic bifurcation nor so high as to be adjacent to the renal arteries (or too far for the access sheath to reach). This chosen crossing spot should then be paired relative to the vertebral body or interdisk space in the same axial cut of the CTA so that it can be identified in the

catheterization laboratory. Typically, crossing happens at the level of the third or fourth lumbar spine. The rationale for avoiding the renal arteries and aortic bifurcation is to preserve the option for use of a covered stent without occluding vital structures. Other aspects of interest on the CTA include the angulation from the IVC to aorta so that appropriate fluoroscopic angles can be used, checking for interposing structures (ie, loops of bowel) between the IVC and aorta, and measuring the diameter of the aorta above and below the intended area of crossing to determine the optimal size of a balloon or covered stent in the event of significant bleeding.

The techniques to gain transcaval access have previously been described (Fig. 4).[40,45] Several key technical considerations are essential to emphasize. Crossing requires electrifying an insulated 0.36-mm (0.014″) wire via electrosurgery pencil connected to the back end. The chosen wire thus must be of reasonably high tip stiffness, and to have a core-to-tip design to transmit the electrical current from the back end of the wire to the tip. The authors typically use an Astato XS 20 wire (Asahi Intecc, Irvine, CA), although multiple manufacturers make wires of this description. Of relevance, most such wires have a polytetrafluoroethylene (PTFE) coating that is electrically insulating. If the wire coating extends all the way through the back end of the wire, the PTFE on the last centimeter of the wire needs to be scrapped off circumferentially with a blade to ensure effective contact between the electrosurgery pencil and wire core. During the subsequent wire crossing process, it is also important to avoid buckling the tip of the wire (Fig. 5) while the electrosurgery pencil is on because this can create a linear laceration along the buckled portion of the tip. Telescoping catheters are then used to introduce a 0.89-mm (0.035″) Lunderquist wire (Cook Medical, Bloomington, IN) over which the large-bore catheter is delivered. Occasionally, the aortic wall requires ballooning before the telescoping microcatheters will cross. The authors typically use a 2.0 × 20-mm compliant balloon across the aortic wall, which is well tolerated (Fig. 6), although, anecdotally, balloons as large as 4.0 mm have been successfully used. Given their length, such balloons are likely to dilate the IVC channel as well.

Following the planned procedure, transcaval closure typically involves placing a nitinol occluder device, typically an Amplatzer ductal occluder 1 (ADO1) (Abbott Vascular, Santa Clara, CA) across the aortotomy. Since the initial

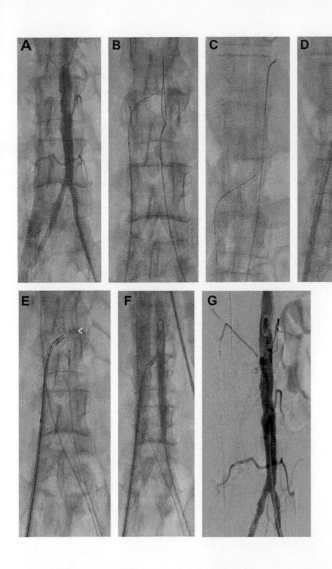

Fig. 4. Fluoroscopic images from a transcaval access procedure, including initial angiography (A), electrified wire crossing into the abdominal aorta from the IVC (B), snaring of the IVC to aortic wire to facilitate delivery of the telescoping microcatheters into the abdominal aorta (C), large-bore sheath delivery across the transcaval access route (D), initial deployment of the Amplatzer Duct Occluder 1 (ADO1; Abbott Vascular, Irvine, CA) (white arrowhead) following completion of the procedure (E), aortography showing patent aorta-IVC fistula before complete deployment of the ADO1 (F), and completion digital subtraction aortography following complete deployment (before release) of the ADO1 (G).

trial, specific technique refinements have been identified to improve hemostasis, and these include ensuring complete reversal of anticoagulation before attempting closure, consistent use of slightly oversized closure devices (typically the ADO1 10/8 mm for transient access, such as during TAVR, and the ADO1 12/10 mm device for indwelling sheaths where less arterial recoil may be expected), the use of a steerable guide (eg, DiRex from Boston Scientific or Agilis from Abbott Vascular) to deflect the closure device horizontally relative to the aorta during deployment, and more liberal use of balloon aortic tamponade with a 1:1-sized compliant balloon inflated for 3 to 5 minutes at a time.

In the setting of MCS, the authors have successfully closed transcaval sheaths left in place for as long as 28 days without complication. In this setting, the sheath must be attached to a continuous flush while in situ and back-bled before removing because the stagnant blood column inside the sheath can clot.

Following occluder device placement, there are 4 general categories of outcomes. The first, which is the least common, is complete occlusion of the aortotomy. The second and most common is a patent caval-aortic fistula without extravasation. The third outcome involves a patent fistula with a cruciform pattern of bleeding into the retroperitoneum. The last possible outcome is complete extravasation from the aorta into the retroperitoneal space. The last 2 scenarios are the most infrequent, and typically are remedied by serial balloon tamponade and, rarely, the use of covered stents. In the original prospective trial of transcaval access, 8 total covered stents were placed; however, these procedures predated the refinements described earlier, and an 8% covered stent rate is far greater than is seen in contemporary practice.[39]

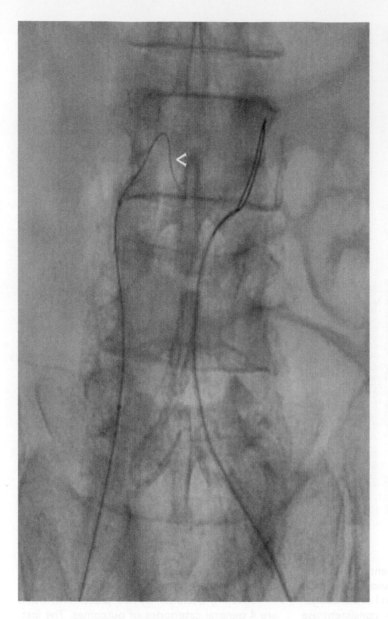

Fig. 5. Fluoroscopic example of a buckled crossing wire deflected off of aortic wall calcium. The white arrowhead indicates the deflected wire.

Caval-aortic fistulas are generally very well tolerated and are typically thought to close over the proceeding days to weeks as the nitinol occluder thromboses. Very recently, the 1-year outcomes of the initial transcaval registry were published showing no cases of late occluder fracture or migration and only 1 caval-aortic fistula still patent in a patient with a grossly misplaced aortic occlusion device.[42]

With more than 1000 transcaval procedures now performed worldwide, transcaval techniques, particularly regarding aortic closure, have been refined and the first purpose-built closure device (Transmural Systems, Andover,

MA) is in testing with 12 subjects enrolled in the early feasibility study to date. It can therefore be expected that outcomes following transcaval access will continue to improve, although there is no current mechanism for systemic data collection of this real-world practice.

COMPARISON OF ALTERNATIVE ACCESS OPTIONS

Both axillary and transcaval access offer opportunities for percutaneous placement of large-bore sheaths and are therefore naturally compared with one another. As with all

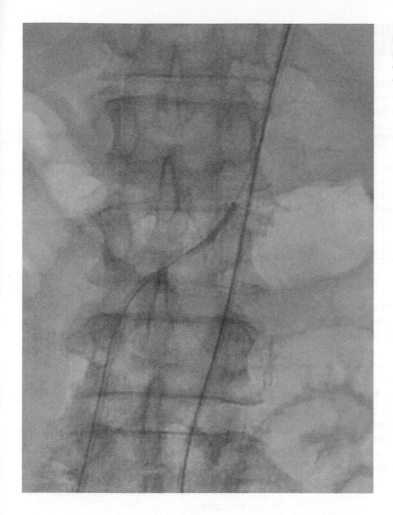

Fig. 6. Fluoroscopic example of ballooning open the aortic wall puncture site to facilitate microcatheter traversal with a 2.0 × 20-mm compliant coronary balloon.

techniques, both options have advantages and disadvantages that should be carefully weighed in the context of each individual scenario (**Table 1**).

The most attractive features of axillary access include patient mobility and opportunities for physical therapy in semidurable implant scenarios (such as with MCS), a generally brief learning curve, the lack of necessary dedicated equipment, the ability to provide manual hemostasis as needed, and the relatively easy corrective actions both percutaneously and surgically should they be required.[27] Further, in cases of long dwell time, such as with MCS devices, the axillary approach may be less prone to infection, as has been shown with central venous catheter placement in this location.[46,47] Alternatively, the axillary artery is not a particularly large vessel in most people[19] and frequently cannot accommodate very large sheaths. Procedural ergonomics and radiation exposure are both worse in axillary

compared with femoral access, although both can be rapidly improved with experience and appropriate room set up. In addition, the potential signal for increased strokes is concerning and requires further evaluation.

Transcaval access also boasts many advantages. Primarily, there are effectively no sheath size restrictions for transcaval access, no potential for ischemia to the limb, and no need for an antegrade perfusion catheter while the sheath is indwelling. In addition, oozing and hematoma around the sheath are rare because the skin puncture is into a femoral vein. Further, procedural ergonomics and radiation exposure are more akin to standard transfemoral procedures. By contrast, limitations with transcaval access include greater procedural cost because of dedicated equipment and a potentially longer learning curve. Complications may be more difficult to remediate because manual-pressure hemostasis is not an option and many

Table 1		
Comparison of transaxillary and transcaval access techniques		
	Advantages	**Disadvantages**
Transaxillary	• Dedicated equipment is not required • Enhanced patient mobility while device indwelling • Short learning curve • Manual hemostasis possible	• Potential for increased exposure to radiation and ergonomic stress with new operators and compared with standard femoral access in general • Smaller caliber of vessel limits sheath size
Transcaval	• No sheath size restrictions • Superficial bleeding/oozing is rare • Ergonomics and radiation exposure comparable with standard femoral access	• Dedicated equipment is required • Remediation of complications can be challenging because of lack of manual pressure options • Bed rest is required; mobility is limited because of indwelling sheaths • Manual hemostasis not possible

interventional cardiologists do not have privileges to stent the aorta. In addition, aortic covered stents themselves often require large-bore arterial access if needed, although, as noted, use of covered stents is significantly down compared with the initial experience, and occlusion balloons can often fit through an 8-French sheath (easily placed in the axillary if the femoral vessels cannot accommodate). In addition, because transcaval access is a form of transfemoral access, bed rest is required in the setting of indwelling sheaths for MCS.

SUMMARY

Structural heart and temporary MCS devices placed via large-bore access continue to evolve. An important part of this growth has been diminishing required sheath sizes. Nevertheless, standard femoral access can be difficult, impossible, or simply the wrong choice for certain clinical scenarios. Innovative options for percutaneous large-bore access exist and are growing in adoption. Both transcaval and axillary access have discrete advantages and disadvantages that can be evaluated in a given clinical scenario. Further collective experience, procedural refinement, and the development of purpose-built devices will continue to improve outcomes for these novel access routes. This article serves as a primer for those operators interested in expanding their practice to include these innovative techniques. However, the worldwide experience with both novel percutaneous access routes is small and much remains unknown. Before initiating a novel access program, operators should consider how frequently they anticipate using these methods, and whether or not other, larger centers within

their regions provide similar services in aggregate. To ensure the best outcomes for their patients, new programs should seek further counsel from a proctor and/or attend a dedicated educational program.

CLINICS CARE POINTS

- Significant iliofemoral peripheral arterial disease can create a barrier to care for patients requiring large bore arterial access.
- Transaxillary or transcaval approaches to vascular access can circumvent this obstacle.
- Specialized training is required to master these techniques.

DISCLOSURES

Dr J.M. McCabe receives honoraria and consulting fees from Abiomed Inc, Boston Scientific, Cardiovascular Solutions Inc, and Edwards LifeSciences. He also reports research funding support from Abiomed Inc.

REFERENCES

1. Mehta SR, Jolly SS, Cairns J, et al. Effects of radial versus femoral artery access in patients with acute coronary syndromes with or without ST-segment elevation. J Am Coll Cardiol 2012;60(24):2490–9.
2. Jolly SS, Yusuf S, Cairns J, et al. Radial versus femoral access for coronary angiography and intervention in patients with acute coronary syndromes (RIVAL): a randomised, parallel group, multicentre trial. Lancet 2011;377(9775):1409–20.
3. Redfors B, Watson BM, McAndrew T, et al. Mortality, length of stay, and cost implications of procedural bleeding after contemporary percutaneous

interventions involving large-bore catheters. J Am Coll Cardiol 2017;69(11):1166.

4. Toggweiler S, Leipsic J, Binder RK, et al. Management of vascular access in transcatheter aortic valve replacement part 1: basic anatomy, imaging, sheaths, wires, and access routes. JACC Cardiovasc Interv 2013;6(7):643–53.

5. Lichtenstein SV, Cheung A, Ye J, et al. Transapical transcatheter aortic valve implantation in humans. Circulation 2006;114(6):591–6.

6. Bleiziffer S, Ruge H, Mazzitelli D, et al. Survival after transapical and transfemoral aortic valve implantation: talking about two different patient populations. J Thorac Cardiovasc Surg 2009; 138(5):1073–80.

7. Cribier A, Durand E, Eltchaninoff H. TAVR, 15 years down shooting for the moon, reaching the stars. J Am Coll Cardiol 2017;70(1):56–9.

8. Grover FL, Vemulapalli S, Carroll JD, et al. 2016 annual report of the Society of Thoracic Surgeons/American College of Cardiology Transcatheter Valve Therapy Registry. J Am Coll Cardiol 2017;69(10):1215–30.

9. Mandawat A, Rao SV. Percutaneous mechanical circulatory support devices in cardiogenic shock. Circ Cardiovasc Interv 2018;10(5):e004337.

10. Metra M, Teerlink JR. Heart failure. Lancet 2017; 390(10106):1981–95.

11. McBride LR, Miller LW, Naunheim KS, et al. Axillary artery insertion of an intraaortic balloon pump. Ann Thorac Surg 1989;48(6):874–5.

12. Bruschi G, Fratto P, Marco FD, et al. The trans-subclavian retrograde approach for transcatheter aortic valve replacement: single-center experience. J Thorac Cardiovasc Surg 2010;140(4):911–5.e2.

13. Schäfer U, Ho Y, Frerker C, et al. Direct percutaneous access technique for transaxillary transcatheter aortic valve implantation "The Hamburg Sankt Georg Approach. JACC Cardiovasc Interv 2012;5(5):477–86.

14. Petronio AS, Carlo MD, Bedogni F, et al. Safety and efficacy of the subclavian approach for transcatheter aortic valve implantation with the corevalve revalving system. Circ Cardiovasc Interv 2010;3(4): 359–66.

15. Modine T, Obadia JF, Choukroun E, et al. Transcutaneous aortic valve implantation using the axillary/subclavian access: feasibility and early clinical outcomes. J Thorac Cardiovasc Surg 2011;141(2):487–91.e1.

16. Mathur M, Krishnan SK, Levin D, et al. A step-by-step guide to fully percutaneous transaxillary transcatheter aortic valve replacement. Structural Heart 2017;1(5–6):209–15.

17. Farhat F, Sassard T, Attof Y, et al. Abdominal aortic aneurysm surgery with mechanical support using the Impella® microaxial blood pump. Interact Cardiovasc Thorac Surg 2008;7(3):524–5.

18. van Mieghem NM, Lüthen C, Oei F, et al. Completely percutaneous transcatheter aortic valve implantation through transaxillary route: an evolving concept. Eurointervention 2012;7(11):1340–2.

19. Arnett D, Lee J, Harms M, et al. TCT-593 caliber and fitness of the axillary artery as a conduit for large-bore cardiovascular procedures. J Am Coll Cardiol 2017;70(18):B245.

20. Tayal R, Iftikhar H, LeSar B, et al. CT angiography analysis of axillary artery diameter versus common femoral artery diameter: implications for axillary approach for transcatheter aortic valve replacement in patients with Hostile aortoiliac segment and advanced lung disease. Int J Vasc Med 2016; 2016:1–5.

21. McCabe J, Khaki A, Nicholson W, et al. TCT-99 safety and efficacy of percutaneous axillary artery access for mechanical circulatory support with the Impella© devices: an initial evaluation from the Axillary Access Registry to Monitor Safety (ARMS) MultiCenter REGISTRY. J Am Coll Cardiol 2017; 70(18):B43.

22. Mathur M, Hira RS, Smith BM, et al. Fully percutaneous technique for transaxillary implantation of the impella CP. JACC Cardiovasc Interv 2016; 9(11):1196–8.

23. Krishnan SK, Mathur M, McCabe JM. Step-by-Step Guide for Percutaneous Transaxillary (PTAX) Transcatheter Aortic Valve Replacment with a Balloon Expandable Valve, the Sapien 3. [Internet]. In: Iribarne A, Stefanescu Schmidt AC, Nguyen TC, 1st eds. American College of Cardiology Transcatheter Heart Valve Handbook: A Surgeons and Interventional Council Review. 2018; Chapter 14, 1–12.

24. Palma RD, Rück A, Settergren M, et al. Percutaneous axillary arteriotomy closure during transcatheter aortic valve replacement using the MANTA device. Catheter Cardiovasc Interv 2018;92(5):998–1001.

25. Yap FY, Alaraj AM, Gaba RC. Inadvertent subclavian arteriotomy closure using the mynx vascular closure device. J Vasc Interv Radiol 2012;23(9): 1253–5.

26. Tayal R, DiVita M, Sossou CW, et al. Efficacy of manual hemostasis for percutaneous axillary artery intra-aortic balloon pump removal. J Interv Cardiol 2020;2020:1–4.

27. Dahle TG, Kaneko T, McCabe JM. Outcomes following subclavian and axillary artery access for Transcatheter Aortic Valve Replacement Society of the Thoracic Surgeons/American College of Cardiology TVT Registry Report. JACC Cardiovasc Interv 2019;12(7):662–9.

28. Gleason TG, Schindler JT, Hagberg RC, et al. Subclavian/axillary access for self-expanding transcatheter aortic valve replacement renders equivalent

outcomes as transfemoral. Ann Thorac Surg 2018; 105(2):477–83.

29. Boll G, Fischer A, Kapur N, et al. Axillary artery conduit is a safe and reliable access for implantation of impella 5.0 microaxial pump. Ann Vasc Surg 2018;48:3–4.

30. Sassard T, Scalabre A, Bonnefoy E, et al. The right axillary artery approach for the impella recover LP 5.0 microaxial pump. Ann Thorac Surg 2008;85(4): 1468–70.

31. Lotun K, Shetty R, Patel M, et al. Percutaneous left axillary artery approach for Impella 2.5 liter circulatory support for patients with severe aortoiliac arterial disease undergoing high-risk percutaneous coronary intervention. J Interv Cardiol 2012;25(2):210–3.

32. Chandrasekhar J, Hibbert B, Ruel M, et al. Transfemoral vs non-transfemoral access for transcatheter aortic valve implantation: a systematic review and meta-analysis. Can J Cardiol 2015;31(12):1427–38.

33. Petronio AS, Carlo MD, Bedogni F, et al. 2-year results of corevalve implantation through the subclavian access a propensity-matched comparison with the femoral access. J Am Coll Cardiol 2012;60(6): 502–7.

34. Jani AR, Blank N, Mohamad T, et al. Axillary artery as alternative access for mechanical circulatory support devices: technique and outcomes from a high volume center. J Am Coll Cardiol 2018;71(11):A1433.

35. Robertis FD, Asgar A, Davies S, et al. The left axillary artery — a new approach for transcatheter aortic valve implantation. Eur J Cardiothorac Surg 2009;36(5):807–12.

36. Laflamme M, Chan L, Mazine A, et al. 507 transcatheter aortic valve implantation via the left axillary artery approach: a single center experience with the medtronic corevalve prosthesis. Can J Cardiol 2012;28(5):S286–7.

37. Truong HD, Hunter G, Lotun K, et al. Insertion of the Impella via the axillary artery for high-risk percutaneous coronary intervention. Cardiovasc Revasc Med 2018;19(5):540–4.

38. Halabi M, Ratnayaka K, Faranesh AZ, et al. Aortic access from the vena cava for large caliber transcatheter cardiovascular interventions pre-clinical validation. J Am Coll Cardiol 2013;61(16):1745–6.

39. Greenbaum AB, O'Neill WW, Paone G, et al. Caval-aortic access to allow transcatheter aortic valve replacement in otherwise ineligible patients initial human experience. J Am Coll Cardiol 2014;63(25): 2795–804.

40. Greenbaum AB, Babaliaros VC, Chen MY, et al. Transcaval access and closure for transcatheter aortic valve replacement a prospective investigation. J Am Coll Cardiol 2017;69(5):511–21.

41. Leon MB, Smith CR, Mack MJ, et al. Transcatheter or surgical aortic-valve replacement in intermediate-risk patients. N Engl J Med 2016; 374(17):1609–20.

42. Lederman RJ, Babaliaros VC, Rogers T, et al. The fate of transcaval access tracts 12-month results of the prospective NHLBI transcaval transcatheter aortic valve replacement study. JACC Cardiovasc Interv 2019;12(5):448–56.

43. McCabe JM. Traversing the chasm transcaval outcomes at 1 year. JACC Cardiovasc Interv 2019; 12(5):457–8.

44. Lederman RJ, Greenbaum AB, Rogers T, et al. Anatomic suitability for transcaval access based on computed tomography. JACC Cardiovasc Interv 2017;10(1):1–10.

45. Lederman RJ, Babaliaros VC, Greenbaum AB. How to perform transcaval access and closure for transcatheter aortic valve implantation. Catheter Cardiovasc Interv 2015;86(7):1242–54.

46. Merrer J, Jonghe BD, Golliot F, et al. Complications of femoral and subclavian venous catheterization in critically ill patients: a randomized controlled trial. JAMA 2001;286(6):700–7.

47. McGee DC, Gould MK. Preventing complications of central venous catheterization. N Engl J Med 2003;348(12):1123–33.

Mechanical Circulatory Support Devices
Management and Prevention of Vascular Complications

Sumit Sohal, MD, Rajiv Tayal, MD, MPH, FSCAI*

KEYWORDS

• Mechanical circulatory support devices • Vascular complications • Prevention

---

KEY POINTS

- The use of mechanical circulatory support devices in acute circulatory collapse and prophylactic high-risk procedures increased by more than 1500% from 2007 to 2011.
- The rate of vascular complications associated with the use of these devices remains between 10% and 16% and are linearly related to increased morbidity and mortality.
- The best method to decrease complications lies in an algorithmic approach, focusing on preventive measures by implementing best practices for vascular access, early recognition, and initiating immediate management techniques for these life-threatening conditions.

INTRODUCTION

Over the last few decades, clinicians have seen gradual development and evolution from simple to more complex and robust mechanical circulatory support (MCS) devices. Since the initial use of the intra-aortic balloon pump (IABP) in the 1960s, several other devices, including extracorporeal membrane oxygenation (ECMO) devices, axial flow pumps such as the Impella and left atrial to femoral bypass systems like Tandem-Heart, are now widely available for use.[1] The world of cardiovascular interventions has not only seen an increase in the indications for these MCS devices, but also a paradigm shift from their use in acute circulatory collapse as in acute myocardial infarction-cardiogenic shock and non–acute myocardial infarction-cardiogenic shock, to the use of these devices in anticipatory or prophylactic fashion in high-risk percutaneous coronary interventions, ablation for arrythmias, and transcatheter valvular interventions.[1,2]

Several studies analyzing the use of devices in the last 2 decades have shown an increasing trend for their use in both acute circulatory collapse and anticipatory use, with Stretch and colleagues[2] reporting an increase of more than 1500% of short-term MCS from 2007 to 2011. These studies also reported a decrease in use of IABPs during the same period, where the use of other peripheral ventricular assist devices (P-VAD; Impella and TandemHeart) and ECMO have increased.[3–6] Shah and colleagues[4] suggested a decrease from 29.8% to 17.7% in the use of IABP from 2005 to 2014, whereas an increase in the use of the Impella and the Tandem-Heart from 0.1% to 2.6% and ECMO from 0.3% to 1.8% during the same time period in patients requiring circulatory support.

TYPES AND TRENDS OF COMPLICATIONS

In current practice, these devices are attractive therapeutic options for our sickest population;

Division of Cardiovascular Diseases, Department of Medicine, RWJ-Barnabas Heath Newark Beth Israel Medical Center, 201 Lyon Avenue, Newark, NJ 07112, USA
* Corresponding author. RWJ-Barnabas Health Newark Beth Israel Medical Center, Suite G4, Newark, NJ 07112.
E-mail addresses: rajtayalmd@gmail.com; rtayal@rwjbh.org

Intervent Cardiol Clin 10 (2021) 269–279
https://doi.org/10.1016/j.iccl.2020.12.008
2211-7458/21/© 2020 Elsevier Inc. All rights reserved.

however, their use has been associated with a myriad of complications. The most common complications are vascular and hematologic; others can be neurologic, infectious, or device-related complications (Box 1).[7,8] Access site or nonaccess site bleeding and acute limb injury are the most dreaded and widely studied complications for MCS devices. Despite an increase in the number of P-VAD implantations and various modifications made in techniques and devices, they require large-bore access and the vascular complications from these continue to be a source of morbidity.[9] In a 10-year US database analysis of P-VADs, after an acute decrease in vascular complications from 21.6% in 2005 to approximately 14.0% in 2006, the rates have not seen a downward trend and have remained steady between 10% and 16%.[8] Bleeding or vascular complications from large-bore access procedures or P-VADs lead to increased length of stay, health care costs, and in-hospital mortality.[8,10]

The rates of the complications are also highly variable among the 4 different types of MCS devices used, with wide ranges reported in various studies.[7] There are no head-to-head trials comparing the complication rates of all 4 MCS devices; however, some studies indicate a trend among these devices. Thiele and colleagues[11] in a meta-analysis compared P-VADs with IABP in

cardiogenic shock, where the use of P-VAD was significantly associated with increased bleeding complications (relative risk, 2.50; 95% confidence interval, 1.55–4.04; P<.001), whereas the rate of leg ischemia was only numerically higher in P-VADs (relative risk, 2.64; 95% confidence interval, 0.83–8.39; P = .10). Karami and colleagues[12] in a study compared Impella with ECMO in patients with cardiogenic shock and reported higher rates of limb ischemia in patients on ECMO as compared with the Impella (5.3% vs 2.2%, respectively). These studies, along with several others, indicate that the lowest rate of bleeding or vascular complications is found with an IABP and the highest with the TandemHeart or ECMO, and may be directly related to increased sheath size and recruitment of sicker population in the later devices.[7,11,12] These findings stress the importance of the prevention and management of these complications to prevent excess morbidity and mortality in these subsets of population.

This article will addresses the vascular complications of the MCS devices and discusses methods for the prevention and management of these complications.

DEFINITION OF VASCULAR COMPLICATIONS

Highly variable rates of complications have been reported from various studies, which is due to a lack of standardized definition of "vascular complications."[7,13] Literature provides standardized definition of these complications for transcatheter aortic valve implantation procedures to define clinical end points in these trials; however, no such definition exist to study MCS devices. Recently, studies have started extrapolating the criteria of defining vascular complications from the Valve Academic Research Consortium to study clinical end points of MCS devices because they also use large-bore arteriotomies.[14–16] The Valve Academic Research Consortium-2 recommends the recording of these complications as access related and non-access related and divides them into major and minor complications (Box 2). This definition also includes the failure of vascular closure devices.[14]

PREVENTION OF VASCULAR COMPLICATIONS

The most important aspect of managing patients with MCS lies in taking preventive measures, identifying early signs of compromise, and

---

Box 1
Tabulated form of various types of complications associated with MCS devices

- Hematologic complications
  - Major bleeding
  - Access site bleeding
  - Thrombocytopenia
  - Hemolysis
  - Thromboembolism
- Neurologic complications
  - Stroke
  - Transient ischemic attack
- Infectious
  - Sepsis
  - Access site infection
- Device related
  - Device migration
  - Device malfunction
- Vascular (see Box 2)

Data from Kappetein AP, Head SJ, Généreux P, et al. Updated standardized endpoint definitions for transcatheter aortic valve implantation: the Valve Academic Research Consortium-2 consensus document (VARC-2)†. *Eur J Cardio-Thoracic Surg* 2012;42(5):S45-S60.

Box 2
Definition of vascular complications as defined by the Valve Academic Research Consortium

Vascular complications (Anyone of the following)

Major vascular complications

- Any aortic dissection, aortic rupture, annulus rupture, left ventricle perforation, or new apical aneurysm or pseudoaneurysm.
- Access site or access-related vascular injury (dissection, stenosis, perforation, rupture, arteriovenous fistula, pseudoaneurysm, hematoma, irreversible nerve injury, compartment syndrome, percutaneous closure device failure) leading to death, life-threatening or major bleeding, visceral ischemia, or neurologic impairment.
- Distal embolization (noncerebral) from a vascular source requiring surgery or resulting in amputation or irreversible end-organ damage.
- The use of unplanned endovascular or surgical intervention associated with death, major bleeding, visceral ischemia, or neurologic impairment.
- Any new ipsilateral lower extremity ischemia documented by patient symptoms, physical examination, and/or decreased or absent blood flow on lower extremity angiogram.
- Surgery for access site-related nerve injury.
- Permanent access site-related nerve injury.

Minor vascular complications

- Access site or access-related vascular injury (dissection, stenosis, perforation, rupture, arteriovenous fistula, pseudoaneurysms, hematomas, or percutaneous closure device failure) not leading to death, life-threatening or major bleeding, visceral ischemia, or neurologic impairment.
- Distal embolization treated with embolectomy and/or thrombectomy and not resulting in amputation or irreversible end-organ damage.
- Any unplanned endovascular stenting or unplanned surgical intervention not meeting the criteria for a major vascular complication.
- Vascular repair or the need for vascular repair (via surgery, ultrasound-guided compression, transcatheter embolization, or stent graft).

Percutaneous closure device failure

- Failure of a closure device to achieve hemostasis at the arteriotomy site leading to alternative treatment (other than manual compression or adjunctive endovascular ballooning).

providing effective management for these vascular complications. These measures, if effectively applied, can help to decrease the mortality, length of stay, and hospital costs associated with these complications. Most of the literature supporting these measures has been studied effectively in patients undergoing transcatheter aortic valve implantation or percutaneous coronary interventions and has been increasingly used in patients requiring MCS devices.[13,17]

The preventive strategies can be divided into preprocedural, intraprocedural, and postprocedural measures and risk factors in each stage can be related to the patient or to the procedure itself. Measures taken in each of these stages can overlap with other stages and should be used to prevent complications.

Preprocedural Preventive Strategies

The most important step in preprocedural prevention is the identification of high-risk patients and undertaking extra precautions in these patients. Several studies have identified patient-related risk factors that lead to high vascular complication rates. Advanced age, female patients, a smaller body surface area, and comorbidities such as diabetes, congestive heart failure, renal failure, and peripheral arterial disease (PAD) are some of the factors that have been associated with high rates of complications and extra vigilance should be applied to these subsets of patients.[7,8,13,16–21]

Preprocedural imaging has a great potential in providing important information before taking the patient to the procedure. Clinical outcomes have improved by the integration of advanced cardiac imaging into planning of percutaneous procedures.[22] Imaging with multidetector computed tomography of the peripheral vasculature can help to calculate the minimal arterial diameter of the femoral artery and identify calcification at the site of possible puncture.[13] Studies have shown that the presence of anterior and posterior calcification may impede the performance of vascular closure devices[23] and that femoral calcification is a predictor of major complications.[21] It is reported that small caliber common femoral and iliac arteries (<5.5 mm) in the setting of PAD combined with large-bore sheaths are associated with increased complications.[9] Hayashida and colleagues[21] and Kadakia and colleagues[20] have proven the importance of calculating the luminal diameter by using the sheath to femoral artery ratio and sheath outer diameter minus minimal artery diameter as predictors of vascular complications, respectively (Fig. 1). These strategies are useful in patients undergoing the prophylactic use of MCS devices in high-risk procedures in planning access sites. An alternate access site such as transaxillary access, transcaval access, or transcarotid access may be considered for use in the event that certain high-risk anatomic features are found in the iliofemoral segment; however, these features may also be limited by a variety of clinical challenges in having well-defined learning curves, requiring specialized equipment, and presenting their own risks for complications.[24] In patients with acute circulatory shock, an immediate decision without preprocedural imaging is often required in contradistinction to those patients undergoing large-bore arterial access for transcatheter aortic valve implantation. In this instance, following an algorithmic approach to access is most beneficial and involves the iterative use of ultrasound assessments before obtaining access, palpation, fluoroscopic identification of major bony landmarks, the use of micropuncture techniques, and iliofemoral angiography after access is obtained or via an alternative access site. This sequence should be implemented into all procedures requiring femoral arterial access procedures because it allows the operator to obtain a tremendous amount of information quickly to make the best appropriate clinical decision for the patient.[9]

The preprocedural treatment of PAD has been used in patients with difficult alternative access and a small minimal arterial diameter of the femoral artery to decrease the risk of vascular complications in these patients. Several studies have been done showing the usefulness of staged procedures in percutaneous procedures.[25–27] The use of regular angioplasty for PAD has not been used frequently in MCS device placement because the increased need for multiple or successive procedures has shown to increase the rate of complications. However, the use of intravascular lithotripsy (IVL), especially in placement of the Impella, insertion has been noted recently. Riley and colleagues[28] described 12 cases of IVL assisted transfemoral Impella insertion, out of which 3 were in cases of circulatory support. This case series shows that IVL can be a valuable adjunct to large-bore access in patients with PAD requiring MCS in both acute and prophylactic scenarios.[28]

Intraprocedural Preventive Strategies
Arterial site access establishment
After careful planning for access site selection, the most important step is establishing arterial site access and sheath insertion techniques. Several ways have been described to decreased higher or lower arterial sticks, both of which are associated with increased vascular complications.[17] The FAUST trial[29] showed that the use of ultrasound guidance for obtaining common femoral artery (CFA) access leads to lesser incidence of large groin hematomas, which was also shown by Elbaz-Greener and colleagues[30] in access for transcatheter aortic valve replacement. Combined ultrasound and fluoroscopy imagining has also been used to gain access to CFA. The use of contralateral side femoral access has also been shown to obtain ipsilateral femoral access, either by using road map approach by doing an angiogram from the opposite site, or by using a J wire from a secondary site to identify the ideal place on the femoral artery and then using ultrasound examination to

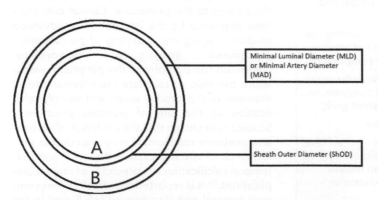

Fig. 1. A sheath inside the vessel. The red line depicts the distance better than the minimal luminal diameter to the sheath outer diameter. These parameters are used to calculate the sheath to femoral artery ratio (SFAR) and sheath outer diameter minus the minimal artery diameter, which have been directly associated with the rate of vascular complications. (A) The sheath. (B) The vessel.

identify the tip of wire and guide the femoral puncture.[13] The use of a micropuncture needle to gain CFA access and then the placement of a sheath over the micropuncture wire, followed by an exchange for a stiff wire and sequential upsizing of dilators before the placement of large sheath is also used as a preventive strategy to avoid complications.[9] The desired angle of access for these procedures is around 45° for femoral access and 30° for axillary access, with the purpose of triangulating the optimal position at which the needle part can be visualized entering the CFA.[31,32] Additionally, a basic ultrasound assessment can also be used in the absence of preprocedural imaging to determine the vessel size, location of the calcification, and disease, and to choose the most suitable point of access. The deployment of 2 Perclose Pro-Glide suture-mediated closure systems is done before upsizing to a large-bore access in the micropuncture technique to facilitate future closure of these large-bore arteriotomies.[9,33,34]

Distal vasculature perfusion
The most dreadful complication associated with large bore sheaths is complete vascular occlusion leading to acute limb ischemia. Several measures have been used to mitigate this vascular complication; however, the cornerstone remains preprocedural anticipation and prevention by obtaining a baseline Doppler ultrasound assessment of the lower extremities and iliofemoral angiography before large-bore sheath insertion, with a quick assessment of distal runoff to the level of the superficial femoral artery. If significant PAD is suspected at this time, it may allow the operator to decide to pursue access in a contralateral limb, an alternative access site, consider the use of IVL, or the preemptive placement of an antegrade perfusion sheath.

i. Peel away sheath: A 2-step peel away sheath design provided by Impella helps to downgrade the sheath size from 14F to 9F and allows for better distal perfusion of the limbs, preventing acute limb ischemia. Precautions should be taken because catheter migration can occur during external sheath removal and can also lead to increased bleeding as the sheath size is tapered down.[9,35,36] Failure to remove the peel away sheath significantly increases the predilection for thrombus formation, regardless of the anticoagulation strategy, although routine sheath flushing protocols have been instituted and may decrease this risk (**Fig. 2**).

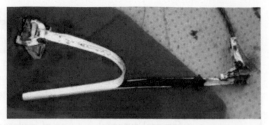

Fig. 2. Thrombus formation in the peel away sheath, reiterating the importance of removing the peel away sheath to prevent clot formation and also helps to improve the distal vascular perfusion.

ii. Bypass procedures: Percutaneous bypass procedures are commonly used to provide distal limb perfusion in large-bore access MCS devices to decrease the incidence of acute limb ischemia. Because the access site can be femoral or axillary in these procedures, bypass procedures have been described for both access sites to provide distal perfusion.[9,37,38] Various techniques are discussed in **Table 1** and **Fig. 3**. **Figs. 4** and **5** shows some of the techniques of femoral bypass (ipsilateral femoral external bypass and contralateral femoral external bypass techniques, respectively) in real-world practice.

iii. Adequate anticoagulation during the procedure prevents thromboembolism and a longer activating clotting time of 200 to 220 seconds is recommended for these bypass procedures.[37]

Postprocedural Preventive Strategies
Frequent monitoring and early recognition of complications
Frequent monitoring of distal extremity pulses clinically and with Dopplers examinations, activating clotting time, and serial biomarker evaluation, such as lactate levels, after the procedure is crucial.[37] The early recognition of clinical symptoms, especially excruciating pain, change in the color of the extremities, decreased urine output, and understanding bedside hemodynamic changes in the MCS device may lead to the prevention of fatal vascular complications.

Arterial access site closure
Site closures should ideally be done in highly controlled settings, such as in a cardiac catheterization laboratory, and not at the bedside to avoid complications.[9] Historically, manual compression has been very frequently used for small-bore access; however, its use in large-bore access sites is controversial because

Table 1
Various strategies available for bypass procedures for distal vascular perfusion in the case of occlusive vascular sheath cutting off the distal blood supply

S. No	Type of Procedure	Description
1	Ipsilateral femoral external bypass	Side arm of large bore sheath is connected to the side arm of the ipsilateral antegrade sheath via a male-to-male connector.
2	Contralateral femoral external bypass	Side arm of contralateral CFA sheath is connected to side arm of ipsilateral antegrade sheath via male-to-male connector
3	Contralateral femoral internal bypass	Side arm of contralateral CFA mother sheath is connected to the side arm of contralateral long 45–55 cm cross-over daughter sheath, which supplies ipsilateral profunda femoris via male-to-male connector.
4	Radial to femoral external bypass	Side arm of radial sheath is connected to the side arm of ipsilateral antegrade sheath via male-to-male connector
5	External axillary radial bypass	Side arm of the large bore sheath is connected to the side arm of the radial sheath.
6	External axillary brachial bypass	Side arm of the large bore sheath is connected to the side arm of the brachial artery via male-to-male connector
7	Internal femoral axillary bypass	Side arm of the femoral mother sheath is connected to the side arm of the daughter sheath which is supplying the ipsilateral brachial artery, via male-to-male connector

bleeding at these sites has led to an increased mortality risk. Although manual compression has been studied for axillary and femoral site closure after IABP removal, alternate suture-based or collagen-based devices have been used for other MCS devices.[15]

i. Vascular closure devices: Suture-based, collagen-based, or hybrid techniques have been frequently used for closing the access sites. The suture-based Perclose ProGuide system has been most frequently used for closure, and its preemptive deployment

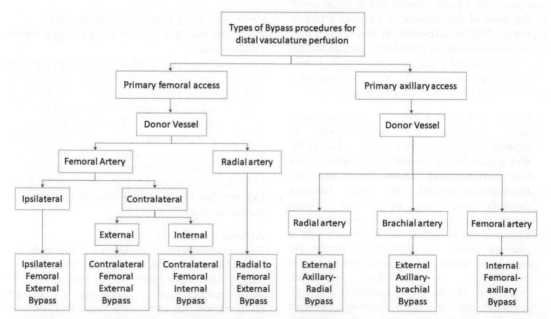

Fig. 3. Flowchart of the various available techniques to provide distal vascular perfusion through bypass procedures.

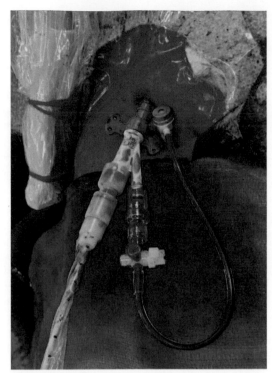

Fig. 4. Real-life picture of an ipsilateral femoral external bypass in which the side arm of a large bore sheath is connected to the side arm of the ipsilateral antegrade sheath via a male-to-male connector.

strategy has been widely used in clinical practice. Another suture-based closure device is the ProStar XL device. A collagen-based device for large-bore access that is widely used is the MANTA; however, some other miscellaneous patch-based (perQseal) or membrane-based (InSeal) devices are

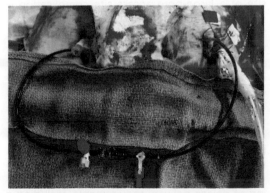

Fig. 5. A real-life picture of a contralateral femoral external bypass in which the side arm of the contralateral CFA sheath is connected to the side arm of the ipsilateral antegrade sheath via a male-to-male connector.

also available; however, they are rarely used. Hybrid techniques use both suture- and collagen-based devices (eg, PerClose and Angioseal) for large-bore arteriotomies have also been studied and used in some centers.[9,33,39,40] The use of 1 method over the other depends on operator experience with a particular device and institution protocol; there are no head-to-head clinical trials comparing the efficacy of one over the other. Familiarity with a post-close technique is also useful when endovascular removal of MCS is needed, especially when the device had been implanted without the concomitant use of a preclose technique. Several techniques are being explored for late closure of large-bore arteriotomies with the MANTA device using ultrasound guidance for depth guard assessment; however, these procedures remain limited by the risk of catastrophic complications. It is important to note that prior publications have shown safety in the delayed deployment of Perclose devices initially placed using the preclose technique without a reported increase in vascular complications or infection and without the routine use of prophylactic antibiotics by maintaining a sterile field and sterilizing the Perclose sutures by using chlorhexidine and separating them from access site by using tegaderm[9,41]

ii. Dry closure technique: This technique, also known as the crossover balloon occlusion technique or temporary endovascular balloon tamponade, has been used by operators to take control of the large-bore access site the during deployment of vascular closure devices to decrease bleeding complications. With this technique, the expansion of a balloon proximal to the large-bore access site advanced from either the contralateral CFA (Fig. 6) or the radial artery (Fig. 7) to temporarily occlude the blood flow in the ipsilateral artery allows the operator to deploy the VSD. Ipsilateral dry closure may also be performed directly through the large-bore sheath and is particularly useful when the single access technique for high-risk percutaneous coronary interventions technique is used (Fig. 8). This process is especially important when, owing to the acuity of procedure, the preclose devices are not deployed preemptively.[9,42,43]

iii. Early bird bleed monitoring system: The first in-human study of an early bird bleed

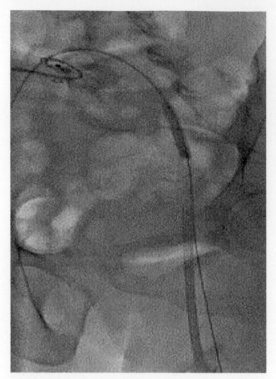

Fig. 6. The technique for dry closure, in which the balloon expanded proximal to the large bore access site is advanced from the contralateral side.

monitoring system, which analyzes bioimpedance, showed positive results in detecting bleeds in patients undergoing endovascular procedures in periprocedural and immediate postprocedure periods and results were comparable with the CT-guided detection of bleeding. However, the use of this device is currently limited and

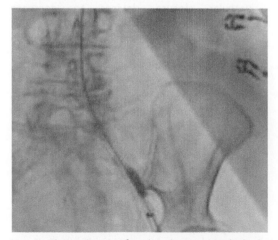

Fig. 7. The technique for dry closure, in which the balloon expanded proximal to the large bore access site is advanced from the radial access site.

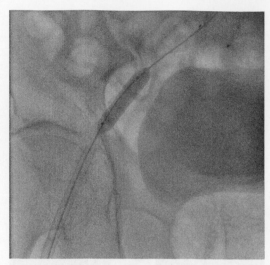

Fig. 8. The technique for dry closure, in which the balloon expanded proximal to the large bore access site is advanced from the ipsilateral side.

not widely studied or used in clinical practice.[44]

MANAGEMENT OF COMPLICATIONS

The most common vascular complications are bleeding from the access site, dissection or perforation of the arteries, retroperitoneal hemorrhage, limb ischemia, and pseudoaneurysm formation.

Cross-Over Technique and Cover Stents

Most of the complications related to access site bleeding, retroperitoneal bleeding, dissection, or perforation of the arteries can be dealt with via a cross-over technique or with a modified cross-over technique in which the ipsilateral site of a large-bore access site complication is examined and managed by accessing it from the contralateral side or from the radial site, respectively.[45,46] Usually, balloon inflation may sometimes suffice; however, self-expandable or balloon-expandable cover stents may be deployed at the site of complications to control it.[47,48] Emergent vascular surgery may be required in some cases where percutaneous procedures do not work; however, these events are becoming more infrequent as operators gain technical endovascular savviness. Essential to this framework becomes a baseline understanding of device delivery requirements, including a knowledge of the device shaft length, stiffness, and sheath size requirements for delivery, because some of these complications can lead to catastrophic collapse within seconds.

Pseudoaneurysm Treatment

Pseudoaneurysms may form at the site of access and may present as a palpable mass with pain and swelling. Most of these masses may thrombose on their own and may not require any treatment; however, some may require ultrasound-guided injection of thrombin into the pseudoaneurysm or stent graft placement. Those that are at a high risk for rupture or may lead to distal ischemia require surgical treatment.[49,50]

Limb Ischemia

Limb ischemia is a dreaded complication that may lead to the loss of the limb and can be life threatening for the patients. The ischemia may occur owing to either occlusion of the vessel, thus cutting off the blood supply, or owing to thromboembolization, especially during sheath removal. Some cases of collagen embolization from closure devices have been noted, leading to ischemia.[51] Prevention and early recognition are the mainstays of management; however, when it happens primary endovascular revascularization, catheter-guided thrombolysis or a combination of both techniques have been described to save the limb.[50]

SUMMARY

MCS devices are increasingly used for acute circulatory collapse or prophylactic high-risk interventions; however, their use is associated with several complications. Vascular complications are associated with increased risk of mortality, hospital stay and costs for patients. The most important strategies to managing these complications are in using preventive strategies at each stage of the procedure, frequent monitoring, early recognition, and immediate intervention to mitigate the effects of these complications.

CLINICS CARE POINTS

- Preventive measures to avoid vascular complications starts with appropriate patient selection and individualizing the treatment strategies according to individual patient characteristics.
- Arterial access establishment and closure are considered most important steps in the use of these MCS devices.
- Strategies to provide distal vascular perfusion should be preemptively planned because

---

acute limb ischemia can be life and limb threatening.

- The choice of vascular closure devices should be individualized from patients' characteristics and operators' experience perspective to provide best results.
- Eventually, early recognition and immediate management should be the key to avoid patient harm from these complications.

REFERENCES

1. Rihal CS, Naidu SS, Givertz MM, et al. 2015 SCAI/ACC/HFSA/STS clinical expert consensus statement on the use of percutaneous mechanical circulatory support devices in cardiovascular care: endorsed by the American Heart Association, the Cardiological Society of India, and Sociedad Latino America. J Am Coll Cardiol 2015;65(19):e7–26.

2. Stretch R, Sauer CM, Yuh DD, et al. National trends in the utilization of short-term mechanical circulatory support: incidence, outcomes, and cost analysis. J Am Coll Cardiol 2014;64(14):1407–15.

3. Panhwar MS, Gupta T, Karim A, et al. Trends in the use of short-term mechanical circulatory support in the United States – an analysis of the 2012 – 2015 national inpatient sample. Struct Heart 2019;3(6): 499–506.

4. Shah M, Patnaik S, Patel B, et al. Trends in mechanical circulatory support use and hospital mortality among patients with acute myocardial infarction and non-infarction related cardiogenic shock in the United States. Clin Res Cardiol 2018;107(4): 287–303.

5. AA P, SJ A, CJ P, et al. The evolving landscape of Impella use in the united states among patients undergoing percutaneous coronary intervention with mechanical circulatory support. Circulation 2020; 141(4):273–84.

6. Khera R, Cram P, Lu X, et al. Trends in the use of percutaneous ventricular assist devices: analysis of national inpatient sample data, 2007 through 2012. JAMA Intern Med 2015;175(6):941–50.

7. Subramaniam AV, Barsness GW, Vallabhajosyula S, et al. Complications of temporary percutaneous mechanical circulatory support for cardiogenic shock: an appraisal of contemporary literature. Cardiol Ther 2019;8(2):211–28.

8. Patel N, Sharma A, Dalia T, et al. Vascular complications associated with percutaneous left ventricular assist device placement: a 10-year US perspective. Catheter Cardiovasc Interv 2020; 95(2):309–16.

9. Kaki A, Blank N, Alraies MC, et al. Access and closure management of large bore femoral arterial access. J Interv Cardiol 2018;31(6):969–77.

10. Redfors B, Watson BM, McAndrew T, et al. Mortality, length of stay, and cost implications of procedural bleeding after percutaneous interventions using large-bore catheters. JAMA Cardiol 2017; 2(7):798–802.

11. Thiele H, Jobs A, Ouweneel DM, et al. Percutaneous short-term active mechanical support devices in cardiogenic shock: a systematic review and collaborative meta-analysis of randomized trials. Eur Heart J 2017;38(47):3523–31.

12. Karami M, den Uil CA, Ouweneel DM, et al. Mechanical circulatory support in cardiogenic shock from acute myocardial infarction: Impella CP/5.0 versus ECMO. Eur Heart J Acute Cardiovasc Care 2019;9(2):164–72.

13. Roberto S, DMG L, Jubin J, et al. Impact of complications during transfemoral transcatheter aortic valve replacement: how can they be avoided and managed? J Am Heart Assoc 2019;8(18):e013801.

14. Kappetein AP, Head SJ, Généreux P, et al. Updated standardized endpoint definitions for transcatheter aortic valve implantation: the valve academic research consortium-2 consensus document (VARC-2)†. Eur J Cardiothorac Surg 2012; 42(5):S45–60.

15. Tayal R, DiVita M, Sossou CW, et al. Efficacy of manual hemostasis for percutaneous axillary artery intra-aortic balloon pump removal. J Interv Cardiol 2020;2020:8375878.

16. Johannsen L, Mahabadi AA, Totzeck M, et al. Access site complications following Impella-supported high-risk percutaneous coronary interventions. Sci Rep 2019;9(1):17844.

17. Bhatty S, Cooke R, Shetty R, et al. Femoral vascular access-site complications in the cardiac catheterization laboratory: diagnosis and management. Interv Cardiol 2011;3(4):503–14.

18. Yatskar L, Selzer F, Feit F, et al. Access site hematoma requiring blood transfusion predicts mortality in patients undergoing percutaneous coronary intervention: data from the National heart, lung, and blood institute dynamic registry. Catheter Cardiovasc Interv 2007;69(7):961–6.

19. Généreux P, Webb JG, Svensson LG, et al. Vascular complications after transcatheter aortic valve replacement: insights from the PARTNER (Placement of AoRTic TraNscathetER Valve) trial. J Am Coll Cardiol 2012;60(12):1043–52.

20. KM B, HH C, DN D, et al. Factors associated with vascular complications in patients undergoing balloon-expandable transfemoral transcatheter aortic valve replacement via open versus percutaneous approaches. Circ Cardiovasc Interv 2014; 7(4):570–6.

21. Hayashida K, Lefèvre T, Chevalier B, et al. Transfemoral aortic valve implantation: new criteria to predict vascular complications. JACC Cardiovasc Interv 2011;4(8):851–8.

22. Blanke P, Weir-McCall JR, Achenbach S, et al. Computed tomography imaging in the context of transcatheter aortic valve implantation (TAVI)/transcatheter aortic valve replacement (TAVR): an expert consensus document of the society of cardiovascular computed tomography. JACC Cardiovasc Imaging 2019;12(1):1–24.

23. Ruge H, Burri M, Erlebach M, et al. Access site related vascular complications with third generation transcatheter heart valve systems. Catheter Cardiovasc Interv 2020. https://doi.org/10.1002/ccd.29095.

24. CA E, MJ M. Alternative percutaneous access for large bore devices. Circ Cardiovasc Interv 2019; 12(6):e007707.

25. Unzué L, García E, Teijeiro R, et al. Transcatheter aortic valve implantation in patients with arterial peripheral vascular disease. Rev Esp Cardiol (Engl Ed) 2017;70(6):510–2.

26. Nascimbene A, Azpurua F, Livesay JJ, et al. Transcatheter aortic valve implantation despite challenging vascular access. Tex Heart Inst J 2015; 42(2):144–7.

27. Ruparelia N, Buzzatti N, Romano V, et al. Transfemoral transcatheter aortic valve implantation in patients with small diseased peripheral vessels. Cardiovasc Revasc Med 2015;16(6):326–30.

28. Riley RF, Kolski B, Devireddy CM, et al. Percutaneous Impella mechanical circulatory support delivery using intravascular lithotripsy. JACC Case Rep 2020;2(2):250–4.

29. Seto AH, Abu-Fadel MS, Sparling JM, et al. Real-time ultrasound guidance facilitates femoral arterial access and reduces vascular complications: FAUST (Femoral Arterial Access With Ultrasound Trial). JACC Cardiovasc Interv 2010;3(7):751–8.

30. Elbaz-Greener G, Zivkovic N, Arbel Y, et al. Use of two-dimensional ultrasonographically guided access to reduce access-related complications for transcatheter aortic valve replacement. Can J Cardiol 2017;33(7):918–24.

31. Dawson K, Jones TL, Kearney KE, et al. Emerging role of large-bore percutaneous axillary vascular access: a step-by-step guide. Interv Cardiol 2020;15: e07 (London, England).

32. Sandoval Y, Burke MN, Lobo AS, et al. Contemporary arterial access in the cardiac catheterization laboratory. JACC Cardiovasc Interv 2017;10(22): 2233–41.

33. van Wiechen MP, Ligthart JM, Van Mieghem NM. Large-bore vascular closure: new devices and techniques. Interv Cardiol 2019;14(1):17–21 (London, England).

34. Toggweiler S, Leipsic J, Binder RK, et al. Management of vascular access in transcatheter aortic valve

replacement: part 1: basic anatomy, imaging, sheaths, wires, and access routes. JACC Cardiovasc Interv 2013;6(7):643–53.

35. Abaunza M, Kabbani LS, Nypaver T, et al. Incidence and prognosis of vascular complications after percutaneous placement of left ventricular assist device. J Vasc Surg 2015;62(2):417–23.

36. Burzotta F, Trani C, Doshi SN, et al. Impella ventricular support in clinical practice: collaborative viewpoint from a European expert user group. Int J Cardiol 2015;201:684–91.

37. Kaki A, Alraies MC, Kajy M, et al. Large bore occlusive sheath management. Catheter Cardiovasc Interv 2019;93(4):678–84.

38. Lichaa H. The "lend a hand" external bypass technique: external radial to femoral bypass for antegrade perfusion of an ischemic limb with occlusive large bore sheath - A novel and favorable approach. Catheter Cardiovasc Interv 2020. https://doi.org/10.1002/ccd.29187.

39. Amponsah MK, Tayal R, Khakwani Z, et al. Safety and efficacy of a novel "hybrid closure" technique in large-bore arteriotomies. Int J Angiol 2017; 26(2):116–20.

40. WD A, Zvonimir K, Janarthanan S, et al. Pivotal clinical study to evaluate the safety and effectiveness of the MANTA percutaneous vascular closure device. Circ Cardiovasc Interv 2019;12(7):e007258.

41. Minha S, Waksman R, Satler LP, et al. Learning curves for transfemoral transcatheter aortic valve replacement in the PARTNER-I trial: success and safety. Catheter Cardiovasc Interv 2016;87(1):165–75.

42. Zaman S, Gooley R, Cheng V, et al. Impact of routine crossover balloon occlusion technique on access-related vascular complications following transfemoral transcatheter aortic valve replacement. Catheter Cardiovasc Interv 2016;88(2):276–84.

43. Genereux P, Kodali S, Leon MB, et al. Clinical outcomes using a new crossover balloon occlusion technique for percutaneous closure after transfemoral aortic valve implantation. JACC Cardiovasc Interv 2011;4(8):861–7.

44. Généreux P, Nazif TM, George JK, et al. First-in-human study of the saranas early bird bleed monitoring system for the detection of endovascular procedure-related bleeding events. J Invasive Cardiol 2020;32(7):255–61.

45. Buchanan GL, Chieffo A, Montorfano M, et al. A "modified crossover technique" for vascular access management in high-risk patients undergoing transfemoral transcatheter aortic valve implantation. Catheter Cardiovasc Interv 2013;81(4):579–83.

46. Sharp ASP, Michev I, Maisano F, et al. A new technique for vascular access management in transcatheter aortic valve implantation. Catheter Cardiovasc Interv 2010;75(5):784–93.

47. Sedaghat A, Neumann N, Schahab N, et al. Routine endovascular treatment with a stent graft for access-site and access-related vascular injury in transfemoral transcatheter aortic valve implantation. Circ Cardiovasc Interv 2016;9(8). https://doi.org/10.1161/CIRCINTERVENTIONS.116.003834.

48. Schahab N, Kavsur R, Mahn T, et al. Endovascular management of femoral access-site and access-related vascular complications following percutaneous coronary interventions (PCI). PLoS One 2020;15(3):e0230535.

49. Ahmad F, Turner SA, Torrie P, et al. Iatrogenic femoral artery pseudoaneurysms–a review of current methods of diagnosis and treatment. Clin Radiol 2008;63(12):1310–6.

50. Tsetis D. Endovascular treatment of complications of femoral arterial access. Cardiovasc Intervent Radiol 2010;33(3):457–68.

51. Goyen M, Manz S, Kröger K, et al. Interventional therapy of vascular complications caused by the hemostatic puncture closure device angio-seal. Catheter Cardiovasc Interv 2000;49(2):142–7.

Moving?

Make sure your subscription moves with you!

To notify us of your new address, find your **Clinics Account Number** (located on your mailing label above your name), and contact customer service at:

Email: journalscustomerservice-usa@elsevier.com

800-654-2452 (subscribers in the U.S. & Canada)
314-447-8871 (subscribers outside of the U.S. & Canada)

Fax number: 314-447-8029

Elsevier Health Sciences Division
Subscription Customer Service
3251 Riverport Lane
Maryland Heights, MO 63043

*To ensure uninterrupted delivery of your subscription, please notify us at least 4 weeks in advance of move.

Printed and bound by CPI Group (UK) Ltd, Croydon, CR0 4YY

03/10/2024

01040374-0018